Tai Chi Walking for Seniors

An Illustrated 4-Week Exercise Program for Fall Prevention, Stronger Balance, Better Health and Daily Confidence in Just 10 Minutes

Xian Ming

Disclaimer

This book is intended for general informational and educational purposes only. The exercises and guidance contained in this publication are not a substitute for professional medical advice, diagnosis, or treatment. Always consult your physician or qualified healthcare provider before beginning any new exercise program, particularly if you have a pre-existing medical condition, recent injury, or surgery.

The author and publisher assume no responsibility for any injury, loss, or damage incurred as a result of the use or application of information contained in this book.

Dedication

For every person who has ever been told, by circumstance, by pain, or by the quiet voice of doubt, that their body is no longer capable of something beautiful.

It is.

This book is for the student who showed up on a Tuesday morning not knowing why, and found something worth returning to. For the hands that shook on the first day and steadied by the fourth week. For the bodies that have carried decades of living and still, every single morning, choose to keep moving.

And for those who loved someone enough to place this book in their hands.

May every page remind you that gentleness is not weakness, that slowness is not failure, and that ten quiet minutes given to yourself each day is one of the most courageous things a person can do.

This is for you.

Table of Contents

A Word Before You Begin

This book was written for the person who hesitated on the top step this morning. The one who reached for the wall without thinking about it. The one who turned down a walk with a friend not because they did not want to go, but because something quiet in the back of their mind said it was better not to risk it.

I have spent fifteen years teaching Tai Chi to older adults in community centers, rehabilitation units, and village halls. I have sat across from hundreds of people at the start of a new program, and I know that particular hesitation well. It is not weakness. It is what happens when a body has given someone a fright, and the nervous system has decided, reasonably enough, that caution is safer from now on.

What I have also seen, again and again, is what happens when that caution begins to lift. Not because someone pushed past it, but because they found a way to move that felt genuinely safe. In the feet. In the hips. In the breath. And when that happens, something changes that goes well beyond the physical.

That is what this program is for.

You do not need any equipment. You do not need previous experience with Tai Chi. You need ten minutes a day and a willingness to pay attention to what your body is doing while you move.

Read this book in order the first time through, especially Chapters 1 through 5. Those chapters are not filler. They are the reason the four weeks of practice actually work. And when you are ready to begin, bring curiosity rather than expectation. Notice what you feel. That noticing is not a warm-up for the real work. It is the real work.

Your first step is the one you take when you turn this page. Take it slowly. That is already the practice.

Xian Ming

Introduction: Walking Changed Everything

Who This Book Is For

There is a particular moment I have heard described more times than I can count. A person is walking across a parking lot, or down a hallway, or across the living room to answer the phone. Their foot catches, or the floor is slightly uneven, or nothing happens at all except that for one half second they are not quite sure they are steady. They catch themselves. Nothing falls. Nobody sees. But something shifts.

From that moment, walking is different. It carries a weight it did not carry before.

This book is for the senior who has started thinking about their feet in a way they never had to before. The one who chooses the chair closest to the wall at a restaurant. Who takes the stairs one at a time now, hand on the rail, when they used to take them without thinking. Who has not fallen, or who has fallen once and will do nearly anything not to fall again.

If any of that sounds familiar, you are in exactly the right place.

Why Walking Got Dangerous

Walking is the most natural thing a human body does. Infants spend their entire first year of life determined to do it. By the time most of us reach adulthood, we do it without giving it a single thought. Thousands of steps a day, completely automatic.

That automaticity is also its weakness.

When balance starts to change, as it does for most people at some point in their senior years, the body's automatic systems begin to lose the fine-tuned precision they once had. The inner ear becomes slightly less reliable. Reaction times slow by measurable fractions of a second. The small stabilizing muscles in the ankles and hips that make constant micro-corrections with every step begin to weaken from underuse. And the nervous system, which once handled all of this without any conscious input at all, starts to ask for help it never needed before.

None of this is catastrophic on its own. Each change is small. But they compound each other, and the result is a body that is no longer quite as confident on its feet as it once was. Falls among older adults are the leading cause of injury-related death and disability worldwide, according to the World Health Organization. In the United States, roughly one in four adults aged sixty-five and older falls each year, according to the Centers for Disease Control and Prevention. In the United Kingdom, the National Health Service reports that falls account for over 250,000 hospital admissions annually among older adults.

These are not numbers about frail people who were already unwell. Many of them are people who were walking perfectly well the day before.

The reason most seniors do not address this proactively is simple: nobody gives them a practical way to do it. Doctors say "be careful." Well-meaning family members suggest slowing down. None of that changes what is actually happening in the body. It just adds anxiety to an already uncertain situation.

This program does something different. It gives you a specific, daily, ten-minute practice that directly trains the systems responsible for balance, stability, and confident movement. Not by working harder, but by working with more attention and intention.

What This Program Does

Tai Chi Walking does four things that most conventional exercise programs for seniors do not.

First, it slows movement down deliberately. This is not a concession to aging. It is a training strategy. Moving slowly forces the nervous system to stay engaged throughout the entire arc of each step, rather than handing control back to automatic pilot the moment a movement becomes familiar. That sustained attention is what rebuilds the fine-tuned balance responses the body has quietly lost.

Second, it trains weight transfer directly. The moment just before a foot lifts, when the full body weight has to shift cleanly from one side to the other, is where most falls actually begin. Tai Chi Walking practices this moment hundreds of times across a session, making it reliable rather than something the body stumbles through.

Third, it uses breath as an active tool. Controlled breathing during movement activates the parasympathetic nervous system, which reduces the tension and physical bracing that make movement stiff and unpredictable. A body that is breathing well moves better. The research on this is consistent and has been for decades.

Fourth, it builds body awareness. Seniors who know where their weight is, where their feet are making contact with the ground, and what their posture is doing in real time are simply less likely to fall. That awareness is trainable, and this program trains it from Day One.

A 2012 study published in the Journal of the American Geriatrics Society found that a twelve-week Tai Chi program reduced fall risk in older adults by 43 percent compared to a stretching control group. A 2017 meta-analysis of ten randomized controlled trials involving more than 2,800 participants, published in the British Journal of Sports Medicine, concluded that Tai Chi significantly reduced both the rate of falls and the number of people who fell. These are not soft findings. They are among the most replicated results in the field of senior fall prevention.

This four-week program will not give you twelve weeks of results in four. But it will give you a genuine foundation. Real changes in how you shift your weight. Real improvement in how your feet meet the ground. A noticeable shift in how walking feels day to day.

How to Use This Book

Read Chapters 1 through 5 before you begin the four-week program. They are not long, and they carry information that will make a direct difference to how much you get out of every session. Chapter 1 explains what is actually happening in your body when balance changes. Chapter 2 explains why Tai Chi Walking addresses it. Chapters 3 and 4 prepare you practically, covering everything from footwear to your own anatomy. Chapter 5 teaches you the core movements before the weekly program asks you to use them.

Chapters 6 through 9 are your four weeks of daily practice. Each chapter covers one week, with a full session structure, movement instructions, and a self-check at the end.

Chapter 10 addresses specific health conditions, including arthritis, osteoporosis, Parkinson's disease, and walking with assistive devices. If any of those apply to you, read that chapter before you begin Week 1.

At the back of the book is the 10-Minute Daily Practice Companion, a week-by-week visual guide designed to sit flat beside you during your sessions so you never need to search for a page while you are trying to move.

One practical note on pacing. Aim for five days of practice each week, not seven. Your body needs two rest days to adapt to what you are asking of it. Mid-morning, somewhere between nine and eleven, works well for most people. By then the stiffness of waking has eased, and the fatigue of the day has not yet arrived. If mornings do not suit you, any consistent time is better than the perfect time you never quite find.

The repetitions listed throughout this book are ranges, not requirements. If I suggest four to six repetitions and three feels like enough today, three is your number. Never argue with your joints.

Chapter 1 begins on the next page. It answers the question most seniors have before they ever begin a balance program, but rarely ask out loud: why is this happening to me?

Chapter 1: Why Your Balance Is Not What It Was

How Balance Erodes with Age

Most people assume that when balance starts to go, it goes all at once. One day you are fine, the next you are not. That is rarely how it happens. Balance erodes gradually, over years, through small and almost invisible changes that pile on top of each other until the body reaches a threshold where ordinary movement suddenly feels less certain than it used to.

Understanding this process is not about accepting decline. It is about knowing exactly what you are working with, and why this program addresses it as precisely as it does.

Your body's ability to stay upright depends on three separate systems working together simultaneously. The first is your vestibular system, housed in the inner ear, which detects changes in your head position and sends rapid signals to your brain about which way is up and how fast you are moving. The second is your visual system, which gives the brain constant reference points in the environment and confirms whether the ground beneath you is level. The third is your proprioceptive system, a network of sensory receptors embedded in your muscles, joints, tendons, and the soles of your feet, which reports on where every part of your body is positioned in space at any given moment.

All three systems operate at the same time. They cross-check each other's signals constantly. When the information from one system is unclear or slightly delayed, the other two compensate. This is a beautifully engineered redundancy, and for most of our lives it works so well we never notice it is happening.

As the body ages, each of these systems changes. Not catastrophically, but measurably. The vestibular system processes signals slightly more slowly. Visual acuity decreases, peripheral vision narrows, and the brain becomes less efficient at using visual input for rapid postural adjustment. Proprioceptive sensitivity in the feet and ankles, which is particularly vulnerable to the effects of reduced circulation and long-term underuse, diminishes in a way that is rarely noticed until a person steps onto an uneven surface and feels genuinely uncertain where their foot has landed.

The result is a body that is still entirely capable of walking safely, but that needs more from you than it used to. It needs conscious engagement. It needs attention. It needs exactly the kind of deliberate, slow, focused movement this program provides.

The Fear-Avoidance Trap

There is a phenomenon well documented in clinical research that is sometimes called the fear-avoidance cycle, and it is responsible for more preventable falls than almost any physical change in the body.

It works like this. A senior has an unsteady moment, a near-miss, or an actual fall. As a direct result, they begin to reduce their physical activity. They walk less, move less, avoid situations that feel uncertain. This feels logical. It feels protective. The problem is that reduced movement causes exactly the physical deterioration it was meant to prevent. Muscles weaken. Balance reactions slow further. Confidence drops. And as confidence drops, the fear grows, which leads to further restriction of movement, which leads to further deterioration.

By the time many seniors arrive at a program like this one, they have been living inside this cycle for months or years. The physical changes are real, but so is the layer of anxiety wrapped around every step. Both need to be addressed.

This program addresses both. Not by telling you to push past your fear, because that is neither helpful nor realistic, but by giving you a practice in which every movement is performed within a range that feels genuinely safe to you on that particular day. Safety is built into the structure of Tai Chi Walking from the ground up. You always have one foot on the floor. Weight is never thrown forward. Movements are slow enough that the nervous system has time to process what is happening and respond, rather than scrambling to catch up after the fact.

What most of my students discover, usually somewhere in the second week of a new program, is that once their body starts accumulating experiences of moving safely, the fear begins to recede on its own. Not because they talked themselves out of it. Because the body's nervous system updated its model of what movement feels like.

That is the real work of this program, and it begins the moment you take your first Tai Chi step.

What the Research Shows

The evidence for Tai Chi as a fall prevention intervention is among the strongest in geriatric research. It has been studied in randomized controlled trials, large meta-analyses, and long-term community programs on multiple continents, and the findings are consistent.

A landmark 2012 study published in the Journal of the American Geriatrics Society followed older adults across twelve weeks of Tai Chi practice and found a 43 percent reduction in fall risk compared to a stretching control group. This was not a marginal improvement. It was the kind of result that prompted clinical guidelines in several countries to begin formally recommending Tai Chi as a fall prevention strategy.

A 2017 meta-analysis published in the British Journal of Sports Medicine reviewed ten high-quality randomized controlled trials involving more than 2,800 participants. The analysis found that Tai Chi significantly reduced both the rate of falls, meaning how often people fell, and the number of people who fell at all. The effect was particularly pronounced in programs that met at least twice weekly, but even once-weekly practice produced measurable benefit.

A 2019 review in the journal PLOS ONE examined twenty-seven studies across a combined total of more than 3,000 participants and concluded that Tai Chi outperformed other common balance interventions, including general stretching, resistance training, and multimodal exercise classes, in reducing fall incidence among community-dwelling older adults.

What these studies share is that the Tai Chi practiced in each of them was not high-intensity or gymnastic. It was slow, deliberate, low-impact movement of exactly the kind you will practice in this program. The results were not produced by extraordinary effort. They were produced by consistent, attentive, daily practice.

Precisely what ten minutes a day, five days a week, across four weeks is designed to build.

Why Moving Beats Resting

The instinct to rest when the body feels unsteady is deeply human. Pain and uncertainty trigger a withdrawal response that has served our species well in genuinely dangerous situations. But for most seniors experiencing the early or moderate effects of balance change, rest is one of the least helpful responses available.

Skeletal muscle begins to lose mass at approximately 3 to 8 percent per decade after the age of thirty, a process called sarcopenia, and that rate accelerates meaningfully after the age of sixty. A senior who reduces their walking by even thirty minutes a day can lose measurable lower-limb muscle strength within weeks. The small stabilizing muscles of the ankle, which are the first line of defense against a stumble, are particularly susceptible to deconditioning because they are used almost entirely in the context of movement. Sitting does not maintain them.

The vestibular system, similarly, is a use-dependent system. It maintains its sensitivity through the experience of movement and postural challenge. A person who stops walking on varied terrain, who avoids gentle slopes or uneven surfaces, who stays seated for long portions of the day, is not protecting their vestibular function. They are allowing it to deteriorate faster than it would have otherwise.

None of this is said to create alarm. It is said because understanding it makes the value of this program concrete and personal rather than abstract. Every ten-minute session you complete is not merely exercise. It is a direct signal to your nervous system, your muscles, and your balance organs that they are needed, that they are being used, and that they should maintain themselves accordingly.

The body responds to that signal. In fifteen years of teaching, I have never once seen a student's balance fail to improve when they showed up consistently and moved with attention. Not always quickly. Not always dramatically. But always in the direction of greater steadiness, greater confidence, and greater freedom in daily movement.

That direction is what this program points you toward. Chapter 2 explains exactly how Tai Chi Walking makes it possible.

Chapter 2: What Tai Chi Walking Actually Is

Where It Comes From

Tai Chi, in its complete form, is an ancient Chinese practice with roots stretching back several centuries. Its full name, Tai Chi Chuan, translates roughly as "supreme ultimate fist," and it originated as an internal martial art, a system of combat that relied not on muscular force but on sensitivity, timing, and the precise coordination of body weight. Practitioners learned to yield to incoming force, to redirect rather than resist, and to generate power through relaxed, rooted movement rather than tension.

Over time, the martial applications became secondary for most practitioners, and what remained was the movement itself: slow, flowing, circular, deeply attentive. By the twentieth century, Tai Chi had spread well beyond China, and researchers began to notice something interesting. People who practiced it regularly, particularly older adults, seemed to fall less, move more freely, and report better physical confidence than those who did not.

That observation led to decades of clinical study, and what the research found is that the same qualities that made Tai Chi effective as a martial art, rooted stable stances, deliberate weight shifting, full-body coordination, breath control, and sustained mental attention, are precisely the qualities that protect against falls and build lasting balance.

Tai Chi Walking draws from this tradition without requiring the student to learn a full form or memorize complex sequences. It takes the core principles of Tai Chi movement and applies them to the one activity every senior does every day: walking. The result is a practice that is both immediately accessible and genuinely powerful, because it trains balance exactly where balance is most needed, in the act of moving from one place to another.

What It Trains That Regular Walking Does Not

Most people assume that walking is already good balance training. In a limited sense, that is true. Regular walking maintains a baseline level of lower-limb function and cardiovascular fitness. But ordinary walking, done at a habitual pace, on familiar surfaces, without conscious attention to what the body is doing, does very little to improve the balance systems described in Chapter 1.

The reason is automaticity. Once a movement becomes automatic, the nervous system stops paying close attention to it. It delegates the task to lower brain centers and frees up conscious resources for something else. This is efficient, but it means the balance systems are not being challenged. They are simply being maintained at whatever level they currently operate, which for many seniors has already declined more than they realize.

Tai Chi Walking interrupts automaticity on purpose. By slowing movement down to a pace that cannot be performed without attention, by requiring the practitioner to feel where their weight is at every moment, by coordinating breath with each step, and by introducing movements the body has not practiced before, it forces the nervous system back into active participation. That active participation is what produces improvement.

Specifically, Tai Chi Walking trains three things that ordinary walking does not address in any meaningful way.

The first is conscious weight transfer. In ordinary walking, weight shifts from one foot to the other quickly and unconsciously. In Tai Chi Walking, the shift is performed slowly and completely before any foot lifts from the ground. This trains the one-leg balance phase of each step, which is the moment of highest fall risk, more directly and repeatedly than any amount of regular walking could.

The second is proprioceptive precision. Moving slowly over a deliberate path, with full attention on the soles of the feet and the sensations of the ankle and hip joints, reactivates proprioceptive pathways that habitual movement has allowed to become quiet. Students consistently report that after two or three weeks of daily practice, they can simply feel where their feet are in a way they could not before.

The third is anticipatory postural control. This is the body's ability to prepare for a movement before it happens rather than reacting to it after. Tai Chi Walking, with its emphasis on stillness and intention before each step, directly trains this anticipatory system. The body learns to organize itself in advance of movement rather than scrambling during it.

Why Slowness Is the Point

One of the most common reactions I encounter when seniors first see Tai Chi Walking is mild surprise at how slow it is. Some expect it to feel like exercise. Others worry it will not do much. A few feel mildly self-conscious moving at what seems like an unusual pace.

The slowness is not a concession to physical limitation. It is the mechanism.

When you walk slowly enough that each step requires genuine attention, several things happen simultaneously. The stabilizing muscles of the ankle, knee, and hip are under sustained load for longer than they would be during a normal stride. The brain receives richer proprioceptive feedback because the movement is slow enough to actually perceive. The vestibular system has more time to process positional information. And the breath, which in hurried movement is often held or disrupted, can remain steady and coordinated with the movement itself.

There is also a neurological dimension to slowness that is particularly relevant for balance training. A 2014 study published in Frontiers in Aging Neuroscience found that slow, mindful movement activates the prefrontal cortex, the part of the brain involved in attention and executive control, to a significantly greater degree than faster, automatic movement. That prefrontal engagement is associated with better postural responses, better dual-task performance, which is the ability to balance while simultaneously doing something else like talking or carrying, and a reduction in the freezing responses that cause many seniors to stumble when their attention is divided.

Moving slowly, in other words, is the practice. It is not a step toward the real practice. The slowness is the training.

Why Ten Minutes Is Enough

A common misconception about exercise is that more is always better. For cardiovascular fitness and muscle hypertrophy, frequency and duration matter significantly. For balance retraining, what matters most is consistency and quality of attention.

Ten minutes of genuinely focused Tai Chi Walking practice produces more neurological benefit than forty minutes of distracted movement. The brain adapts to what it is asked to do repeatedly, not to how long it is asked to do it. Short, consistent, high-quality sessions train the nervous system more effectively than long, occasional ones.

The ten-minute structure of this program was not chosen arbitrarily. It reflects the research on motor learning in older adults, which consistently shows that sessions of eight to fifteen minutes, performed five or more times per week, produce faster and more durable improvements in balance and gait than longer sessions performed less frequently. A 2020 study in the Journal of Aging and Physical Activity found that older adults who practiced balance exercises for ten minutes daily showed equivalent postural stability improvements at eight weeks to a group that practiced for thirty minutes three times weekly.

There is also a practical argument that matters just as much as the scientific one. A ten-minute commitment is achievable. It fits before breakfast, between appointments, during a quiet afternoon. It does not require special preparation, a cleared schedule, or a particular level of physical readiness. And because it is achievable, seniors actually do it. Consistency is the variable that most determines outcome in this kind of training, and ten minutes makes consistency possible in a way that longer programs rarely do.

By the end of four weeks, most people find that ten minutes feels natural. Some extend their practice voluntarily. Some simply keep to ten minutes for months or years. Both are entirely valid. The foundation this program builds does not require expansion to remain useful. It simply needs to continue.

Chapter 3 is where the practical preparation begins. Before your first step, there are a few things worth getting right.

Chapter 3: Getting Ready

Talking to Your Doctor First

Before you begin any new physical program, a brief conversation with your doctor or healthcare provider is worth having. This is not about seeking permission. It is about gathering information that will make your practice safer and more effective from the very first session.

The conversation does not need to be long. You are telling your provider that you are starting a gentle, low-impact walking practice that involves slow deliberate movement, weight shifting, and ten minutes of daily activity. You are asking two questions. First, is there anything about your current health, medications, or recent procedures that I should be aware of before I begin? Second, are there any movements I should avoid or modify given my specific situation?

Most seniors will receive a straightforward green light. Some will receive useful guidance about specific joints, blood pressure responses to standing, or medications that affect balance, including certain blood pressure drugs, diuretics, antihistamines, and sleep medications that are known to increase dizziness and fall risk as a side effect. That information is genuinely valuable to have before you start, not after.

A few conditions warrant particular attention. If you have had a recent fracture, joint replacement, or cardiac event, your provider may want to clear you for the specific types of movement involved. If you have peripheral neuropathy, which reduces sensation in the feet and legs, your provider may suggest particular modifications. Chapter 10 covers these conditions in detail, and it is worth reading alongside any guidance your provider gives you.

If you do not have a regular healthcare provider, or if accessing one is difficult, the movements in this program are designed to be safe across a wide range of senior fitness levels. Start with Week 1, keep movements slow and within your comfortable range, always maintain contact with a wall or chair when instructed, and stop if you feel pain, dizziness, or significant shortness of breath. Those are the same principles a thoughtful provider would give you.

What to Wear and Where to Walk

The right clothing and footwear make a meaningful difference to how safe and comfortable your practice feels, and neither needs to be expensive or specialized.

Footwear is the most important consideration. The ideal shoe for Tai Chi Walking has a thin, flat sole with a firm heel counter, the rigid part that cups the back of the foot. This gives you clear feedback through the soles of your feet about where your weight is, which is essential for the proprioceptive training at the heart of this practice. Thick cushioned athletic shoes, despite feeling comfortable, actually reduce ground feedback significantly. Running shoes with a heel drop, where the heel sits higher than the toe, alter your posture and weight distribution in ways that work against the rooted, level stance this program requires.

Good options include flat canvas shoes, thin-soled walking shoes, Tai Chi slippers if available, or any flat shoe with a non-slip sole and a supportive heel. Avoid walking barefoot, particularly on hard floors, as the lack of grip increases slip risk. Avoid thick socks with no shoes for the same reason.

Clothing should be loose enough to allow a full range of hip and knee movement without restriction. Elastic-waist trousers, comfortable joggers, or loose linen trousers work well. Tight jeans, structured trousers, or anything that restricts the hip joint will limit the quality of your weight shift and make the movements feel more effortful than they need to be. A fitted shirt or t-shirt is better than a loose outer layer that you cannot easily see your body through, because part of the practice involves noticing your own posture.

Remove shoes with heels of any kind. Remove slippery socks. Remove anything that restricts ankle movement.

Floor Surfaces and Safe Spaces

Your practice space needs to meet four criteria: non-slip flooring, enough clear space to take four to six steps in a straight line, proximity to a wall or sturdy piece of furniture for moments when support is needed, and reasonable freedom from distraction and clutter.

Non-slip flooring is the most critical. Polished hardwood or tile without a mat is acceptable if clean and dry. Carpet with a low, firm pile is excellent for practice as it provides grip and some cushioning. Loose rugs are the single most dangerous element in any home practice space and should be removed or moved before every session, not just remembered as something to step over. They are responsible for a disproportionate number of indoor falls among seniors.

A clear path of four to six steps in a straight line is sufficient for almost all the movements in this program. This can be a hallway, a living room with the coffee table moved slightly, or any open floor area of roughly ten to twelve feet. You do not need a large space.

Keep a sturdy chair or a clear section of wall within arm's reach for the first two weeks, even if you feel confident you will not need it. Having it available changes the quality of your movement. When the body knows support is nearby, it relaxes the bracing tension it holds as a precaution, and relaxed movement is better movement.

Outdoors is a valid practice space from Week 3 onward, once the core movements are comfortable. Chapter 9 addresses outdoor practice specifically. For the first two weeks, indoors on a familiar, predictable surface is recommended.

Using Support Without Shame

I want to address this directly because it comes up almost every time I begin practice with a new group of students.

Using a wall, a chair back, or a cane during practice is not a sign of weakness. It is not a sign that you are not ready. It is not something to graduate out of as quickly as possible. For many seniors, having that support available is precisely what allows them to practice with enough relaxation to actually improve.

The purpose of support in this program is not to hold you up. It is to give your nervous system a safety anchor while it is learning new movement patterns. Think of it the way a child uses a bicycle with training wheels. The training wheels are not doing the balancing. The child is. The training wheels simply prevent the cost of a mistake from being too high while the skill is developing.

There is no movement in this program that cannot be modified to include wall or chair contact. If you need both hands on a chair back for Week 1, that is exactly where you should be. If by Week 3 you find yourself touching the wall only occasionally, that is genuine progress. If you still want that wall nearby in Week 4, that is also entirely valid.

What matters is that you show up, move with attention, and respect what your body tells you on any given day. The support is a tool. Use it as long as it serves you.

Chapter 4 is where we turn the attention fully inward. Before you take your first Tai Chi step, it is worth spending a little time understanding the body that is going to take it.

Chapter 4: Know Your Body Before You Walk

Your Feet and the Ground

Stand up for a moment, if you are able to do so safely. Place your feet flat on the floor, about hip-width apart. Close your eyes if that feels comfortable. Now simply notice what you feel through the soles of your feet.

Most people, when they do this for the first time, are mildly surprised. They feel the texture of their socks, the firmness of the floor, and if they pay close attention, a subtle and constant shifting of pressure across the sole as the body makes hundreds of tiny adjustments to stay upright. That shifting is happening all the time, every moment you stand or walk. The difference between a person with strong balance and one with compromised balance is not whether those adjustments happen. It is how quickly, how accurately, and how completely they happen.

The foot is not simply a platform you stand on. It is one of the most sophisticated sensory organs in the body. The sole of each foot contains a dense concentration of mechanoreceptors, sensory nerve endings that respond to pressure, vibration, and the direction of force. These receptors send continuous information to the brain and spinal cord about the body's relationship to the ground beneath it. When this information is accurate and fast, balance responses are precise. When it is degraded, through reduced circulation, neuropathy, or simply the long-term effect of wearing thick-soled shoes that buffer the foot from ground feedback, balance responses become slower and less reliable.

This is why footwear matters as described in Chapter 3, and it is why much of this program begins and ends with attention to the feet. In almost every session, you will be asked to notice what you feel through your soles. Not to force a sensation, but simply to allow awareness to settle there. That act of attention alone, repeated daily, begins to restore the sensitivity that years of automatic, unattended movement have allowed to dim.

The toes also play a role that is often underappreciated. The big toe in particular acts as a final point of balance leverage, providing a push-off platform and a gripping mechanism on any surface that is not perfectly level. Many seniors have weakened toe flexors from years of sedentary habits or ill-fitting footwear. The movements in this program, with their deliberate heel-to-toe weight transfer and full foot contact at each step, gently strengthen this area without any targeted exercise being required.

Your Hips and Weight Transfer

If the feet are where the body meets the ground, the hips are where the body manages the meeting. The hip joint is the fulcrum of all upright movement. Every step, every shift of weight, every turn of direction involves the hips redistributing the body's mass from one side to the other and then back again.

In ordinary walking, this redistribution happens quickly and largely outside of conscious awareness. In Tai Chi Walking, it is performed deliberately and completely. This is the single most important mechanical distinction between this practice and regular walking, and it is the reason the practice produces such significant improvements in fall prevention.

The technical term for what Tai Chi Walking trains is complete unilateral weight bearing: the ability to shift the full weight of the body onto one leg cleanly and steadily, leaving the other leg entirely free to move. Most falls happen not during the step itself, but during this transition, the brief moment when weight is in the process of transferring and neither foot has full contact. If that transition is rushed, incomplete, or mechanically sloppy, the body is vulnerable.

By practicing this transfer hundreds of times in each session, slowly enough that the stabilizing muscles of the hip abductors, the gluteus medius and gluteus minimus, have time to engage fully, Tai Chi Walking builds the strength and coordination that make this transition reliable. Students who have practiced for even two weeks consistently report that they feel more planted, more planted on the standing leg, more in control of the moving leg, and more aware of the difference between the two.

Your hips will also tell you things during practice that are worth listening to. Tightness in the hip flexors, which is common in seniors who spend significant time seated, will limit the length of your stride and the completeness of your weight shift. The movements in this program do not require a large stride. They require a complete weight shift, and those are different things. Work within the range your hips offer you today. That range will expand as the weeks progress.

Your Spine and Your Center

The spine does two things simultaneously in Tai Chi Walking, and both are essential. It keeps the body upright, and it transmits the rotational movements of the walk from the lower body to the upper body and back again.

Good spinal alignment in this practice means standing tall without being stiff. The image I use with my students is a thread attached to the crown of the head, drawing it gently upward. Not pulling the chin up, which creates tension in the neck. Not arching the lower back, which shifts the weight backward and narrows the base of stability. Simply a gentle lengthening of the entire spine from the tailbone to the crown, with the natural curves of the back preserved rather than flattened or exaggerated.

Many seniors carry significant forward flexion in their posture, a rounding of the upper back called kyphosis, which can develop gradually from years of sitting, from osteoporosis affecting the vertebrae, or simply from the habitual forward lean that many people unconsciously adopt as a response to feeling less steady on their feet. This forward lean shifts the center of mass forward and ahead of the base of support, which significantly increases fall risk.

Tai Chi Walking does not require you to correct your posture before you begin. It asks you to bring a little more awareness to it with each session. The movements themselves, particularly the Rooted Stance and the Slow Forward Walk, gently encourage better spinal alignment through the physical demands of the practice rather than through instruction alone. Over the four weeks, most students find their posture improving as a natural consequence of the practice, not as a separate effort.

Your center, in Tai Chi terminology, refers to a point approximately two inches below the navel and two inches inward, called the dan tian. This is not a mystical concept. It corresponds closely to the body's actual center of mass, and in Tai Chi practice it is used as a reference point for initiating movement. When movement originates from this central point rather than from the extremities, the body moves as a coordinated whole rather than in disconnected parts. That coordination is part of what makes Tai Chi Walking feel different, and more stable, than ordinary walking.

Your Eyes, Ears, and Balance System

As described in Chapter 1, the vestibular system in the inner ear is one of the three pillars of balance. It detects angular acceleration and linear movement of the head, and it sends signals to the brain and to the muscles of the eyes and neck to keep the visual field stable and the body upright during movement. When the vestibular system is functioning well, all of this happens without any conscious effort. When it is not, movement feels uncertain, and the visual system has to compensate by doing more work.

For most seniors, the vestibular system has not failed. It has simply slowed. The signals it sends are accurate, but they arrive slightly later than they used to, which gives the body slightly less time to respond. The result is not vertigo or spinning, but a mild imprecision in postural responses that adds up to reduced stability over the course of a day.

The eyes contribute to balance in two ways. First, they provide spatial reference points that tell the brain where the body is in relation to the surrounding environment. Second, they participate directly in the righting reflex, the automatic response that corrects a postural disturbance before it becomes a fall. When gaze is fixed, unsteady, or poorly directed, both of these contributions are degraded.

In Tai Chi Walking, you will be guided to keep a soft, forward gaze: not looking at your feet, which pulls the head down and compromises spinal alignment, and not looking far into the distance with a tense, searching focus, but a relaxed, middle-distance awareness that keeps the visual system engaged without creating tension. This quality of gaze, calm and receptive rather than anxious and searching, makes a practical difference to how steady movement feels. You will notice this in the first session.

Breath as Your Anchor

Breathing during movement is one of the most consistently underused tools in senior balance training, and one of the most powerful available.

When the body perceives a threat to its stability, whether that threat is real or anticipated, the stress response activates. Adrenaline rises. Muscles tighten. The breath becomes shallow and held. The diaphragm contracts. Blood flow is redirected away from the extremities. In a genuine emergency, this cascade is useful. In the context of a balance program, it creates the exact conditions that make falls more likely: stiff muscles, reduced proprioceptive sensitivity, and a nervous system operating in alarm mode.

Slow, controlled breathing reverses this cascade. A long, unhurried exhale activates the parasympathetic nervous system, the body's rest-and-recover state, and produces measurable reductions in muscle tension, heart rate, and cortisol within seconds. A body that is breathing well is a body that is relaxed, and a relaxed body moves more freely, more accurately, and more safely than a braced one.

In this program, breath is used as an anchor throughout every session. Each movement is coordinated with either an inhale or an exhale. The timing is not rigid. If you lose track of the breath coordination, simply return to slow, natural breathing and the coordination will reestablish itself. What matters is that the breath is never held, never forced, and never rushed.

One simple practice before every session: stand quietly for thirty seconds, place one hand lightly on your abdomen, and take three slow breaths, feeling the abdomen rise on the inhale and fall on the exhale. This is not a warm-up exercise. It is a signal to the nervous system that what follows is safe, deliberate, and within your control. Every session in this program begins this way.

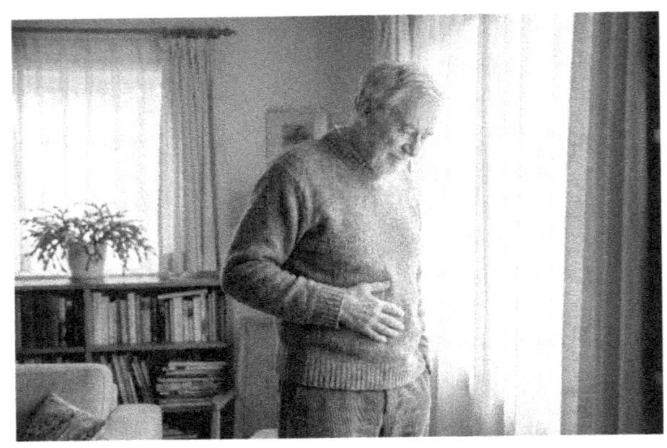

You now have the understanding needed to begin. Chapter 5 is where the movements themselves start. Everything you have read in Chapters 1 through 4 was preparation for this. Take it at whatever pace your body offers today.

Chapter 5: The Core Movements

This chapter is your movement library. The core movements of this program are all introduced here, described fully and illustrated clearly. Read through the entire chapter before you begin Week 1. You do not need to practice all the movements now unless you want to. Simply reading and visualizing each one will give your nervous system a useful first impression before the body is asked to perform.

When the week chapters refer to a movement by name, such as the Empty Step or the Arm Coordination, they are referring to exactly what is described and illustrated here. The weekly sessions will not ask you to use a movement without preparing you for it.

In one or two cases across the four weeks, a new movement may be introduced at a point in the program when the body is genuinely ready for it, rather than before the practice has begun. Where that happens, the reason is given clearly and the instructions for the new movement are made available.

The Rooted Stance

The Rooted Stance is not a step. It is the ground beneath every step. Every session in this program begins and ends here, and you will return to it between movements whenever you need a moment to reset.

How to perform it:

Step 1 — Position your feet

Stand with feet parallel, hip-width apart. Hip-width is roughly the distance between your hip bones, slightly narrower than your shoulders.

Step 2 — Soften your knees

Do not lock your knees straight. Let them release very slightly, just enough to feel a gentle bend.

Step 3 — Relax your arms

Let both arms hang at your sides. Palms face inward toward your thighs. Fingers are loose.

Step 4 — Drop your shoulders

Let your shoulders fall away from your ears. If they feel tight, take a breath in, then let them drop on the exhale.

Step 5 — Lift through the crown

Imagine a gentle upward lift from the very top of your head toward the ceiling. At the same time, let your tailbone drop very slightly downward. This lengthens the spine without stiffening it.

Step 6 — Feel your feet

Bring your attention down to your feet. Feel four points of contact on each foot:

- Base of the big toe
- Base of the little toe
- Inner heel
- Outer heel

Let your weight spread evenly, left and right, front and back.

Step 7 — Take three slow breaths

Breathe in slowly through the nose. Breathe out slowly through the mouth. With each exhale, let the face soften, the jaw unclench, the neck release. Do this three times before you begin any movement.

This is your starting point. Take your time here. There is no movement yet, only arrival.

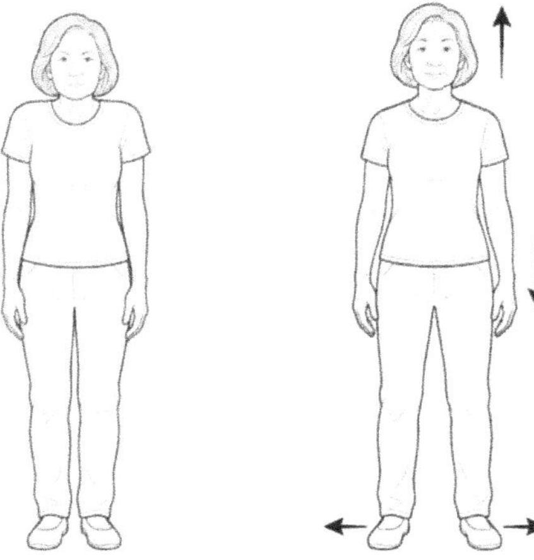

Before: tense stance   **After: rooted stance**

What to feel for: Evenness across both feet. Softness in the knees. Length through the spine without stiffness. Breathe moving freely.

Modification: If standing without support is uncertain, place one hand lightly on the back of a sturdy chair beside you. This does not change the quality of the stance. It simply removes the anxiety that prevents full relaxation.

The Empty Step

The Empty Step is the most important single skill in this entire program. It is the foundation of safe walking, and it is the one movement that most directly addresses fall risk.

An Empty Step is a step in which the foot that is about to move carries no weight before it lifts. The full weight of the body has already shifted completely to the standing leg. The moving foot is entirely free, entirely "empty," before it leaves the floor.

This sounds simple. In practice, most people discover in the first session that they have never actually done this in their ordinary walking. They lift a foot while it still carries a portion of their weight, which is why a stumble or an uneven surface can so easily knock them off balance. If weight is still on the foot that catches, the body has no margin for error.

How to perform it:

Step 1 — Start in the Rooted Stance

Feet hip-width apart, knees soft, arms relaxed at your sides.

Step 2 — Shift your weight to the left foot

Slowly move your entire weight onto your left foot. Feel it press more firmly into the floor.

Step 3 — Feel the right side lighten

As weight leaves the right side, notice the right hip rise very slightly. This is natural and correct.

Step 4 — Lift the right foot

Only when the weight transfer feels complete, lift the right foot just slightly, no more than half an inch off the floor.

Step 5 — Hold and feel

Hold for two seconds. The lifted foot should feel completely weightless, no effort needed to keep it up.

Step 6 — Return and repeat

Place the right foot back down. Now repeat the same sequence on the other side.

That is the Empty Step in its simplest form. The foot that lifts should feel completely light, with no effort needed to hold it up because all the weight has already left it.

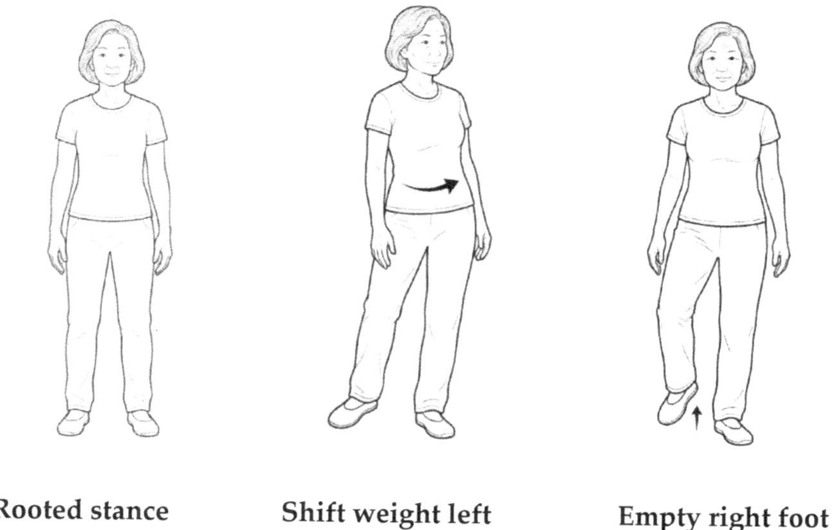

What to feel for: The standing leg feeling solid and fully loaded. The lifting foot feeling genuinely weightless. No wobble in the hips during the transfer.

Modification: Perform with one hand resting on the back of a chair until the weight shift feels reliable on its own.

The Forward Walk

The Forward Walk is the Empty Step set in motion. It is not the walk you already know. It is a deliberate, heel-first, unhurried step that keeps the body completely organized throughout the entire arc of movement.

Step 1 — Start in the Rooted Stance

Feet hip-width apart, knees soft, arms relaxed and hanging at your sides with palms facing inward toward the thighs.

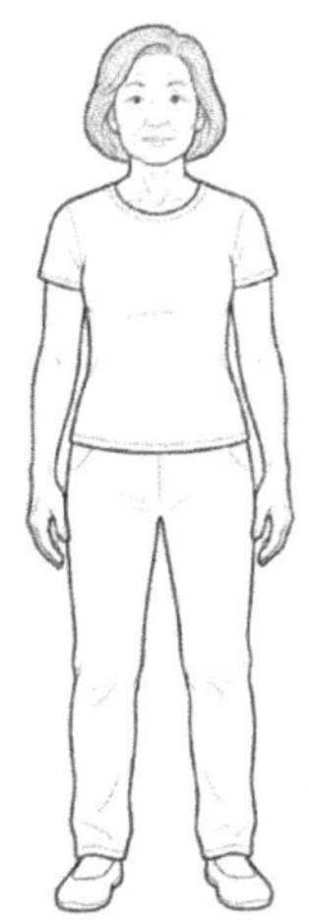

Step 2 — Shift your weight to the left foot

Slowly move your entire weight onto your left foot using the Empty Step. Feel the left foot press more firmly into the floor before anything else moves.

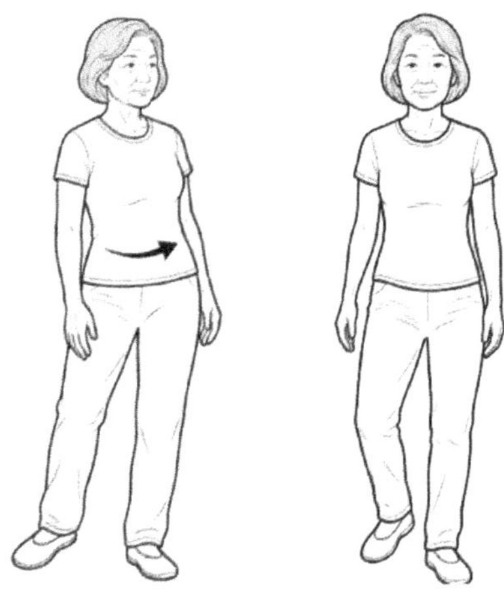

Step 3 — Feel the right side lighten

As weight leaves the right side, notice the right hip rise very slightly. The right foot is now empty and ready to move. Do not rush this moment.

Step 4 — Move the right foot forward

With the right foot completely free, slowly reach it forward. Land the heel first, with intention. Do not let the foot slap down.

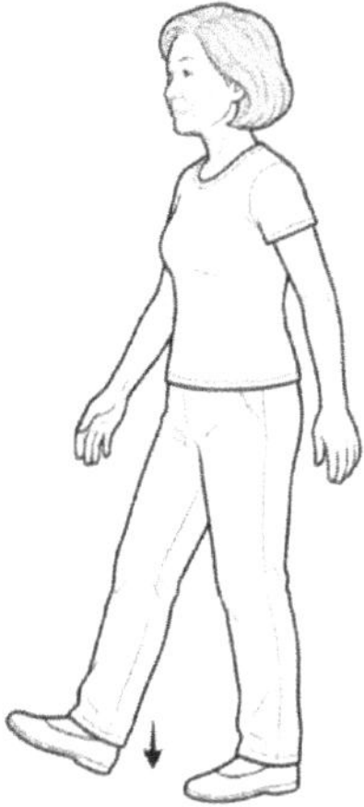

Heel lands first

Step 5 — Roll through the foot

Once the heel makes contact, gradually roll the sole forward until the full foot is flat on the floor — heel, then arch, then ball, then toes.

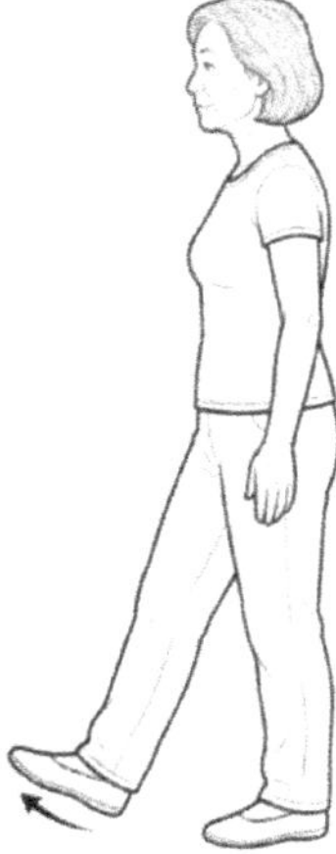

Step 6 — Shift your weight forward onto the right foot

As the right foot lands fully, begin moving your weight forward onto the right leg, travelling through the foot from heel to toe until the right side is fully loaded.

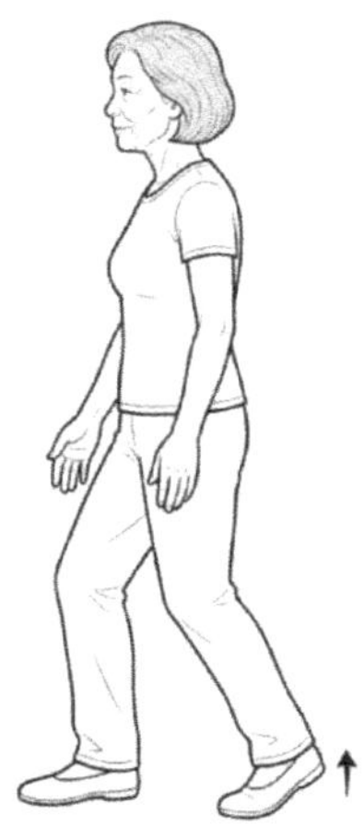

Weight transfers forward

Step 7 — Feel the left side lighten

As weight fully reaches the right side, the left foot becomes empty. Notice it; do not lift it until the transfer is complete.

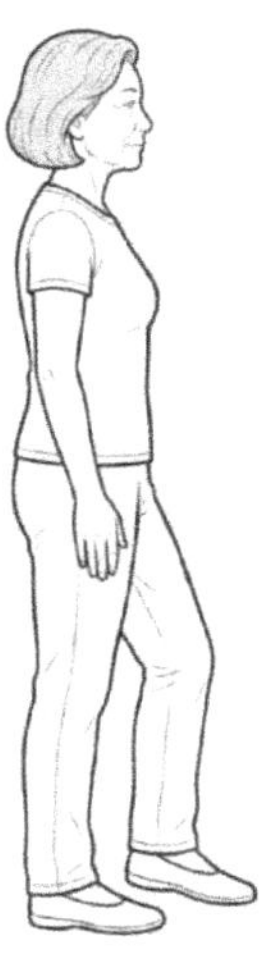

Step 8 — Bring the left foot forward

With the left foot now completely free, slowly reach it forward in the same manner. Heel first, roll through, then shift weight forward. This completes one full cycle of the Forward Walk.

The pace should feel slow enough to be slightly unusual. If it does not feel slow, it is probably not slow enough.

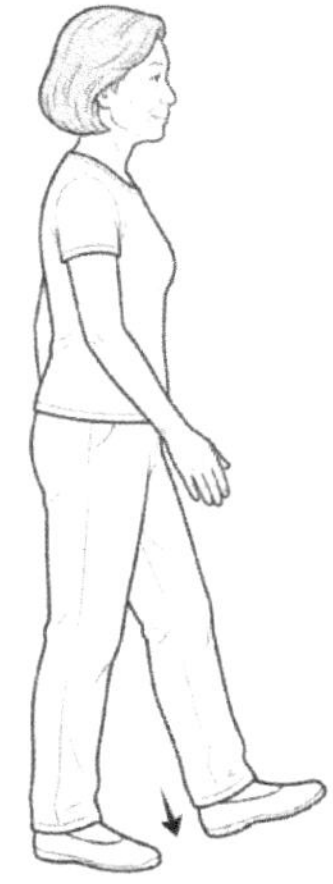

What to feel for: Heel contact before any other part of the foot. The full roll from heel to toe before weight shifts. Complete weight transfer to the front foot before the back foot lifts. No hurrying.

Modification: Take only two steps forward, then pause in the Rooted Stance before continuing. There is no minimum number of steps per sequence.

The Side Step

The Side Step trains lateral balance, the ability to move and stabilize the body on a horizontal plane. Most falls among seniors occur during forward movement, but many of the most dangerous ones happen during a sideways movement, turning to reach something to the side, stepping around an obstacle, or simply shifting direction unexpectedly.

How to perform it:

Step 1 — Start in the Rooted Stance

Feet hip-width apart, knees soft, arms relaxed and hanging at your sides with palms facing inward toward the thighs.

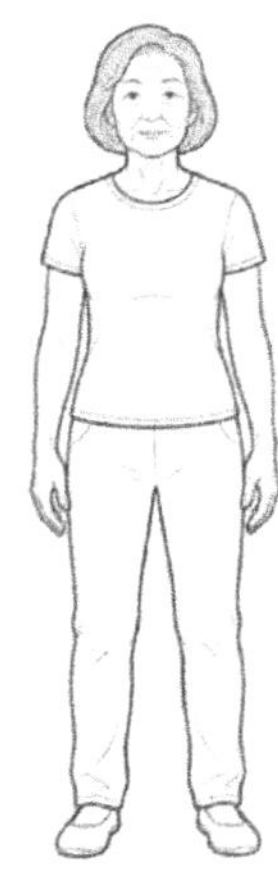

Step 2 — Shift your weight completely to the left foot

Slowly move your entire weight onto your left foot. Feel it press more firmly into the floor. Take your time here. The shift should feel complete and deliberate, not rushed.

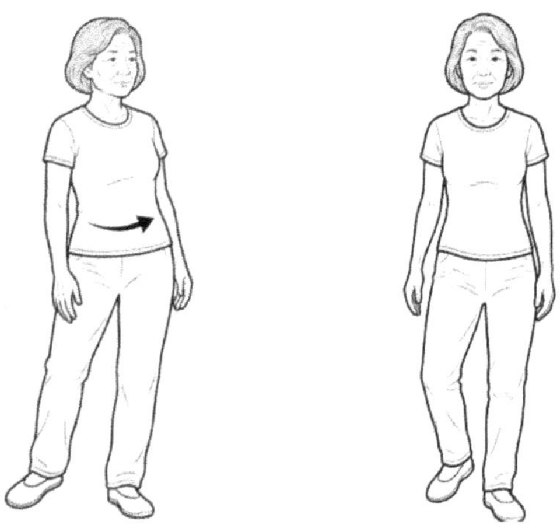

Step 3 — Feel the right side lighten

As weight leaves the right side, notice the right hip rise very slightly. This is natural and correct. The right foot should begin to feel light and free against the floor.

Step 4 — Step the right foot directly sideways

Only when the weight transfer feels complete, lift the right foot just slightly and step it directly out to the right, approximately one foot-width. Place it flat on the floor, not toe-first, not heel-first. The whole sole lands at once.

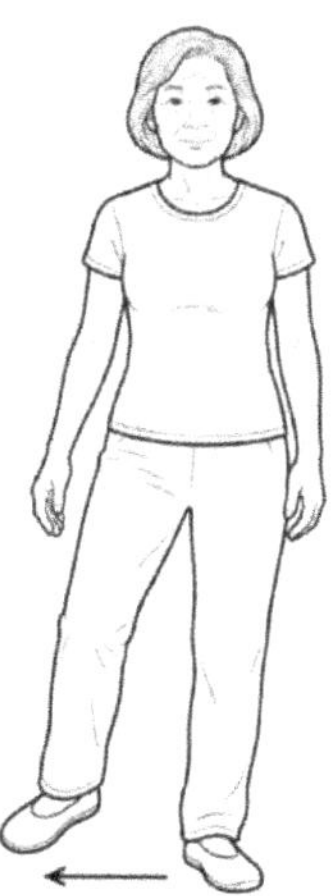

Step 5 — Shift your weight completely to the right foot

Slowly transfer your entire weight across to the right foot. Feel it press firmly into the floor. Let the left side lighten in the same way the right side did in Step 3.

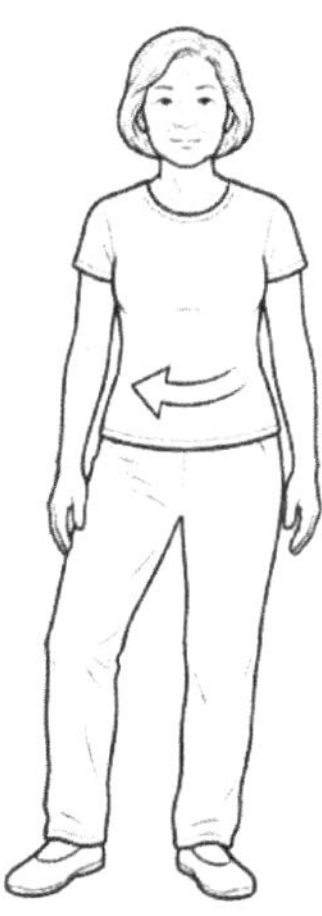

Step 6 — Draw the left foot in to meet the right

6a. When the left foot feels completely empty, lift it just slightly and begin drawing it inward. The left foot lifts free of the floor; heel and toes both off the ground and travels inward toward the right foot.

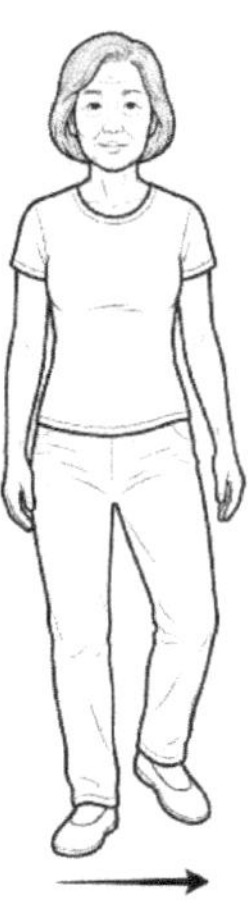

The gap between the feet is still wider than hip-width. The right foot remains firmly planted.

6b. Continue drawing the left foot inward until it lands flat at hip-width.

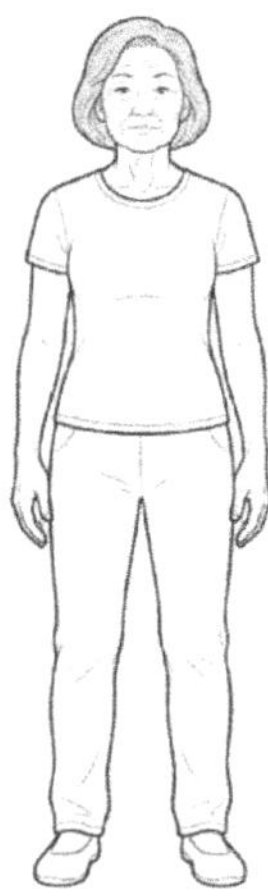

The entire left sole lands flat simultaneously, not heel-first, not toe-first. Both feet are now parallel and hip-width apart. Weight returns equally to both legs. Pause fully at this Rooted Stance position before the next cycle.

Step 7 — Repeat and then reverse

Perform two to three more open-and-close cycles stepping to the right, pausing in the Rooted Stance between each one. Then repeat the full sequence stepping to the left, shifting weight to the right foot first each time.

The key is that the feet never cross. One foot steps out, the other follows to maintain the stance width. This is not a crossing step. It is a controlled lateral open-and-close.

What to feel for: The complete weight shift before the stepping foot lifts. The stepping foot landing flat, not toe-first or heel-first. The drawing foot returning to exactly hip-width, not wider or narrower.

Modification: Perform with one hand on the wall beside you until the lateral weight shift feels dependable.

The Backward Step

Walking backward is one of the most effective balance exercises available to seniors, and one of the most underused. It activates the posterior chain of muscles, the hamstrings, gluteus maximus, and spinal erectors, which are precisely the muscles responsible for preventing a backward fall, the most common direction of falls among older adults.

How to perform it:

Step 1 — Start in the Rooted Stance

Feet hip-width apart, knees soft, spine upright, arms relaxed and hanging at your sides with palms facing inward toward the thighs.

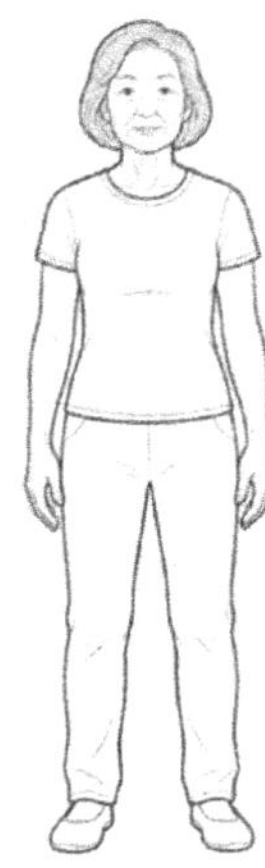

Step 2 — Shift your weight completely to the right foot

Slowly move your entire weight onto your right foot. Feel it press more firmly into the floor. The shift should feel complete and deliberate, not rushed.

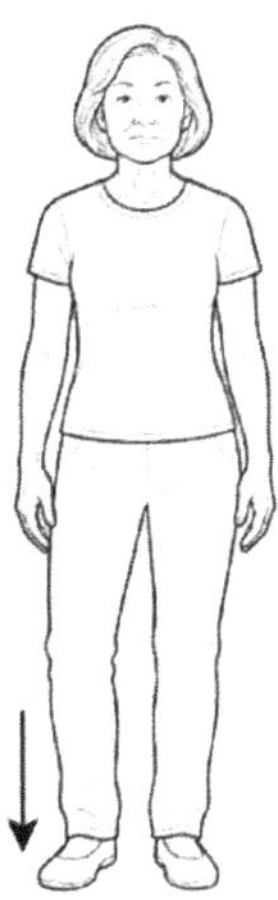

Step 3 — Feel the left side lighten

As weight leaves the left side, the left foot will begin to feel light and free against the floor. Wait until it feels truly empty before moving.

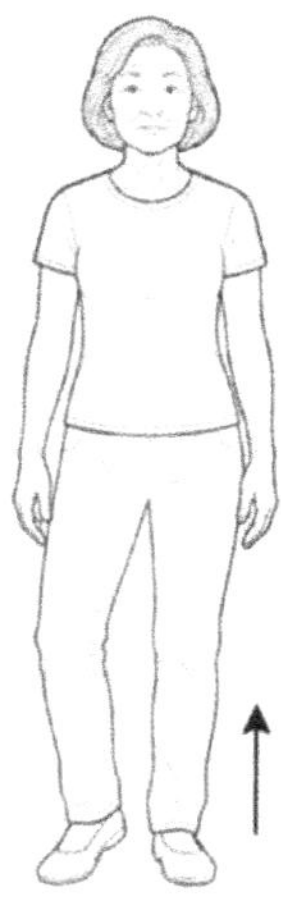

Step 4 — Reach the left foot backward

Slowly reach the left foot backward, placing the toes on the floor first, then gently lowering the heel. This toe-first contact is the reverse of the forward walk earlier discussed.

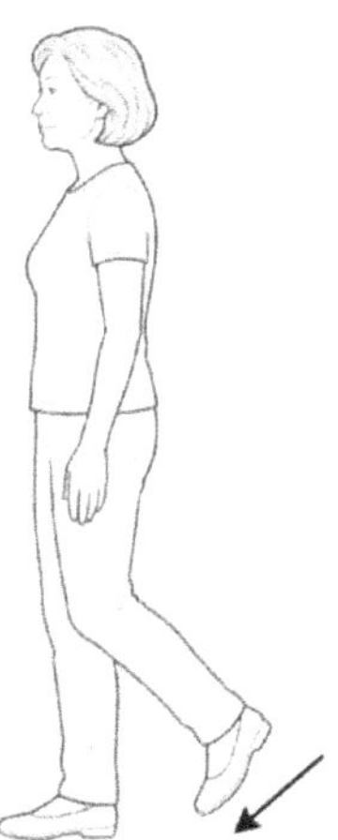

Toes touch first

Step 5 — Shift your weight backward onto the left foot

Once the left foot is flat on the floor, slowly transfer your entire weight onto it. Feel it press firmly into the floor. The right side will begin to lighten.

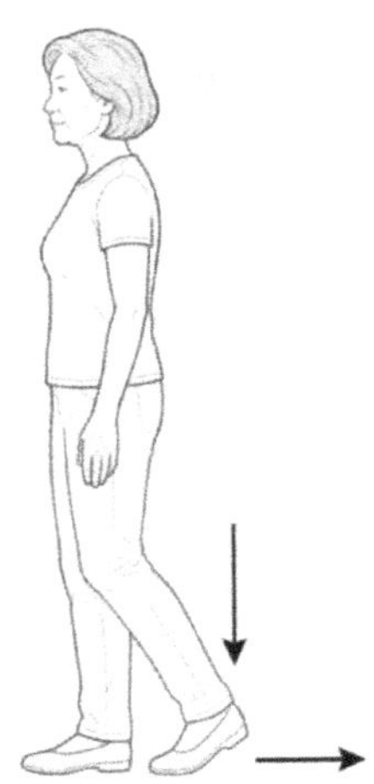

Weight shifts back

Step 6 — Step the right foot back and continue

When the right foot is empty, step it back to meet the movement and continue. Keep the spine upright throughout. Do not lean forward to compensate for the backward direction.

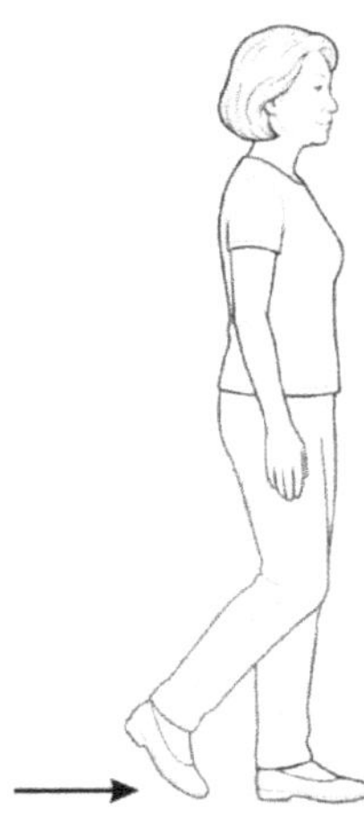

What to feel for: Toes touching first before the heel. The spine staying upright rather than tilting forward. Weight fully transferring to the back foot before the front foot lifts.

Modification: Perform only one backward step at a time, returning to the Rooted Stance between each step. Keep one hand on the wall until the movement feels reliable.

Safety note: Always check that the space behind you is clear before beginning backward steps. A brief glance over one shoulder before starting is sufficient.

The Arm Coordination

The arms in Tai Chi Walking are not passengers. They are active participants that help the body stay coordinated, counter-rotate the torso, and maintain fluid movement through the entire kinetic chain.

In ordinary walking, the arms swing opposite to the legs: when the right leg steps forward, the left arm swings forward, and vice versa. This cross-body pattern is not aesthetic. It is structural. It creates a counterbalancing rotation through the spine that reduces lateral sway and keeps the center of mass stable.

In Tai Chi Walking, the same principle applies, but the arm movement is conscious, deliberate, and coordinated with the breath.

How to perform it:

Step 1 — Start in the Rooted Stance

Feet hip-width apart, knees soft, arms relaxed and hanging at your sides with palms facing inward toward the thighs.

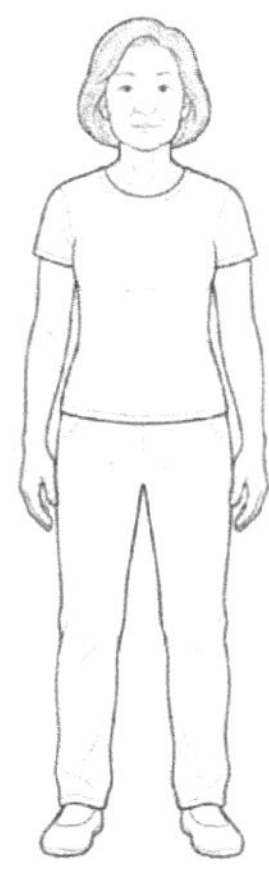

Step 2 — Step forward with the right foot

As your right foot steps forward, let your left arm swing gently forward and your right arm move slightly back. Keep your hand relaxed and open. The swing is small, no wider than your body, no higher than your hip.

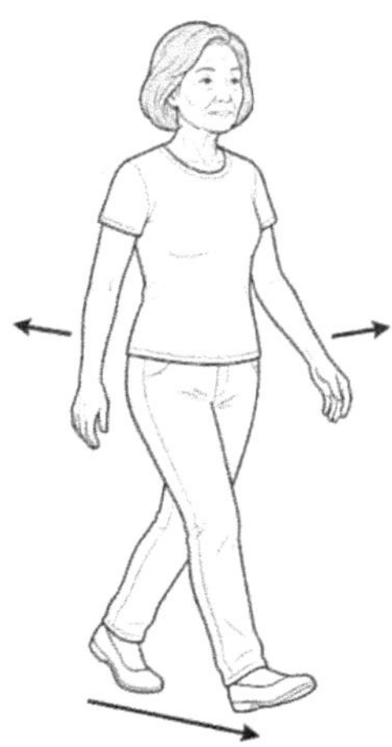

Step 3 — Inhale as the foot steps

Breathe in as the right foot steps forward. Let the breath come naturally with the movement.

Step 4 — Exhale as the weight settles

As your weight moves fully onto the right foot, breathe out. Feel the body soften and the arms loosen slightly.

Step 5 — Step forward with the left foot

Now the left foot steps forward. The right arm swings gently forward and the left arm moves slightly back. Same small, easy swing as before.

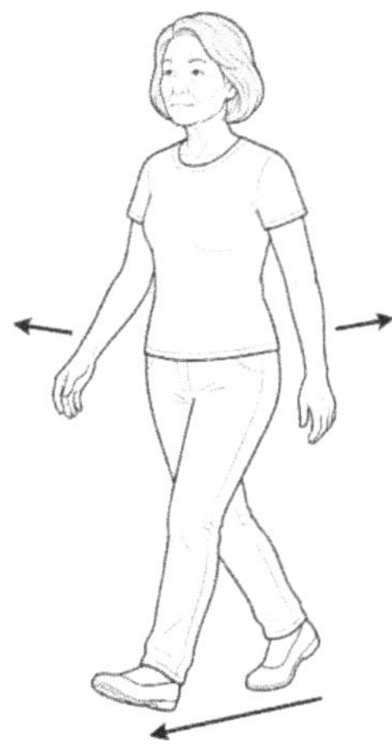

Step 6 — Keep going, one step at a time

Inhale with each step. Exhale as the weight settles. Let the arms follow naturally; opposite arm, opposite leg. After a few steps, it will feel easy and automatic.

What to feel for: The arms feeling relaxed and loose, not stiff or held. The cross-body pattern feeling natural after two or three steps. A slight sense of rotation in the torso with each step.

Modification: Begin with just the forward walk and no arm movement. Add the arm swing only when the weight transfer feels reliable on its own.

You now have the foundation of this program. The movements in this chapter form the base of everything you will practice across the four weeks ahead. In later weeks, one or two new movements are introduced at the moment the body has been prepared enough to receive them, rather than at the start. Nothing will be asked of you before you are ready. Before turning to Week 1, take a moment to simply stand in the Rooted Stance, take three slow breaths, and notice how your body feels today. That act of noticing, right now, before a single week has begun, is already the practice.

Chapter 6: Week 1 — Slow Down to Build Up

What This Week Asks of You

Week 1 asks exactly one thing: that you show up and move slowly.

Not perfectly. Not impressively. Not for long. Just slowly, and with attention, for ten minutes, five days this week.

That is the whole assignment.

I say this because most people arrive at the first week of a new program carrying an internal standard they have not spoken aloud. A sense that they should already be better at this than they are. A quiet frustration when something feels awkward or unfamiliar. A tendency to judge the quality of a session by whether it felt smooth, rather than by whether it happened at all.

In Week 1, none of those standards apply. Awkward is correct. Slow is correct. Uncertain is correct. The nervous system is meeting these movements for the first time with conscious attention, and that process is inherently a little unsteady. A student named Margaret, who came to one of my classes several years ago, described her first week as feeling like she was learning to walk again, but this time actually paying attention. That is a precise description of what Week 1 is.

What you are building this week is not yet visible in how you move. It is happening in the nervous system, in the muscles, in the proprioceptive pathways of the feet and ankles. The foundation is being laid. You will not see it yet. But it is real, and it is cumulative, and by the end of Week 2 you will feel it.

Daily Session Structure

Every session this week, and every session in the weeks that follow, follows the same three-part structure. It never varies because the structure itself is part of the training.

Part 1: Arrive — 2 minutes

Stand in the Rooted Stance. Place one hand on your abdomen if it helps. Take three slow breaths, feeling the abdomen rise and fall. Bring your attention to your feet, then slowly scan upward through the ankles, knees, hips, spine, and shoulders. You are not looking for anything specific. You are simply arriving in your body before you ask it to move. This two-minute arrival practice is not optional. It is what separates a useful session from a mechanical one.

Part 2: Practice — 6 to 7 minutes

Perform this week's movements in the sequence listed below. Take your time between movements. There is no rush to get through the sequence. If you lose your place, return to the Rooted Stance, take one breath, and continue.

Part 3: Close — 1 to 2 minutes

Return to the Rooted Stance. Take three slow breaths. Roll the shoulders gently backward once or twice. Rotate the ankles one at a time in slow circles, four rotations each direction. Then stand still for thirty seconds and notice how your body feels compared to when you arrived. This closing noticing is not an evaluation. It is information.

This Week's Movements

This week introduces four movements from Chapter 5. They are performed in the order listed. Read the full description in Chapter 5 for each movement before your first session. During the session itself, use the brief cues below.

Movement 1: The Rooted Stance

Use at the start, between movements, and at the close of every session.

Stand with feet hip-width apart, knees soft, spine long. Four corners of each foot on the floor. Shoulders dropped. Breathe moving freely. Hold for three breaths before beginning any movement.

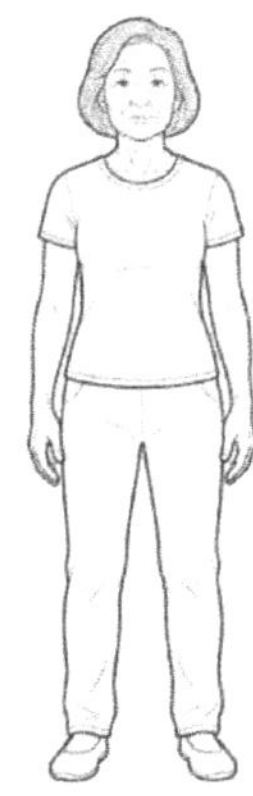

Perform at the start and close of every session, and as a reset point between Movement 2, Movement 3 and Movement 4.

Movement 2: The Empty Step

Performed in place, not traveling forward yet.

From the Rooted Stance, shift your weight fully to the left foot. When the right foot feels completely light, lift it just slightly off the floor. Hold for two seconds.

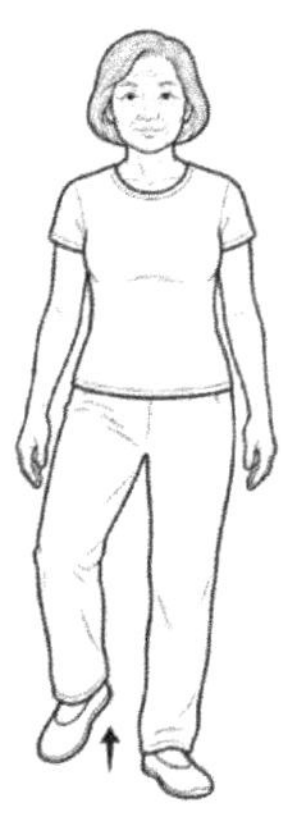

Empty right foot

Replace it. Shift weight fully to the right foot. Lift the left foot slightly. Hold for two seconds. Replace it. That is one cycle.

- **Repetitions:** 4 to 6 cycles per session
- **Rest:** Return to Rooted Stance for two breaths between every two cycles
- **Support:** One hand on chair back if needed, throughout

This movement trains the single most important balance skill in the program: complete weight transfer before any foot leaves the floor. Do not rush the shift. The shift is the exercise.

Movement 3: The Forward Walk

Traveling forward, heel first, slowly.

From the Rooted Stance, perform the Empty Step to free the right foot, then step it forward, landing heel first.

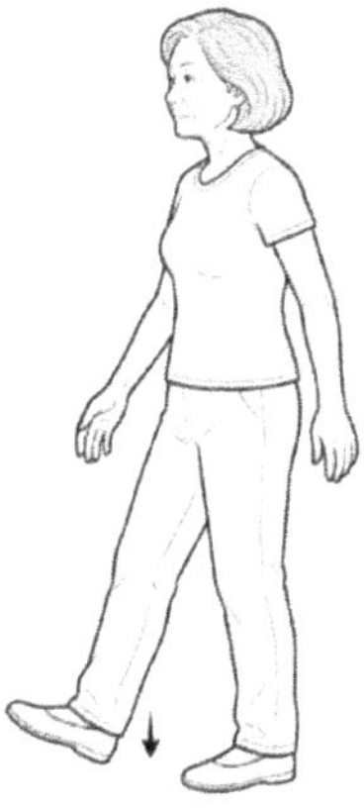

Heel lands first

Roll slowly through the heel to the toe. Shift weight forward.

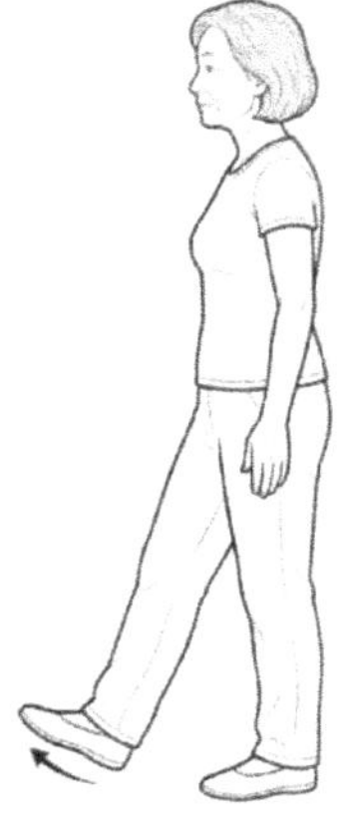

Roll slowly

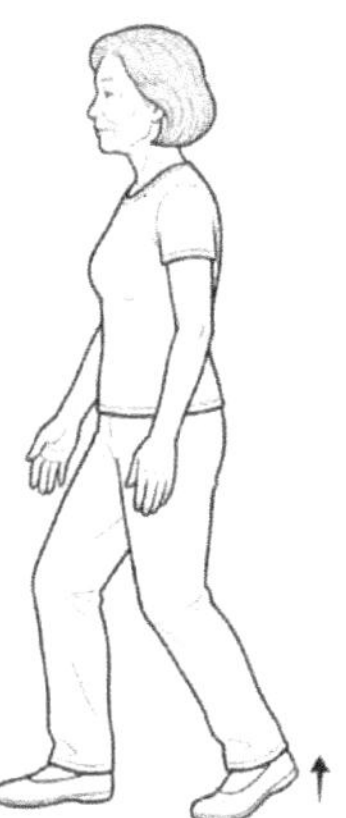

Weight transfer to right foot

Free the left foot and step forward in the same way. Walk forward for four to six steps, then turn around using small steps and return. That is one pass.

- **Repetitions:** 3 to 4 passes per session
- **Rest:** Pause in Rooted Stance for two breaths between passes

    Note: A pass is one complete walk from one end of your practice space to the other end; and the reverse counts as a second pass and so on.

- **Support:** Walk alongside a wall with fingertips lightly touching if needed
- **Pace:** If it does not feel slightly slower than necessary, slow down further

Movement 4: Forward Walk with Arm Coordination

Only begin this movement once Movement 3 feels settled, not earlier than Day 3 of this week. Do not add the arms on Day 1 or Day 2. The weight transfer needs to feel reliable first before the arms are introduced.

From the Rooted Stance, begin the Forward Walk exactly as in Movement 3 above.

As the right foot steps forward, let the left arm swing gently forward and the right arm move slightly back.

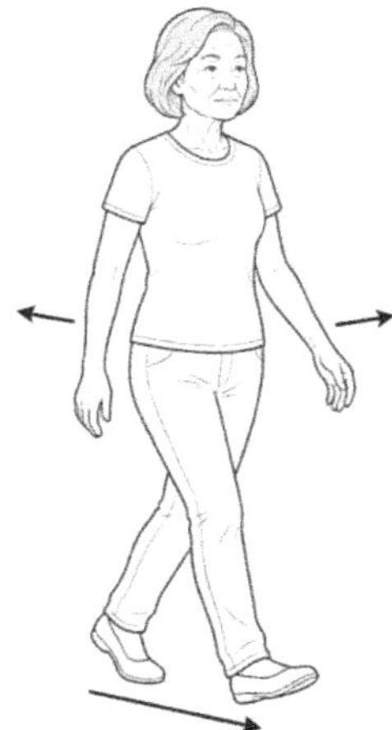

As the left foot steps forward, the right arm swings forward and the left moves back. The swing is small, no wider than the body, no higher than the hip. Hands are relaxed and open throughout.

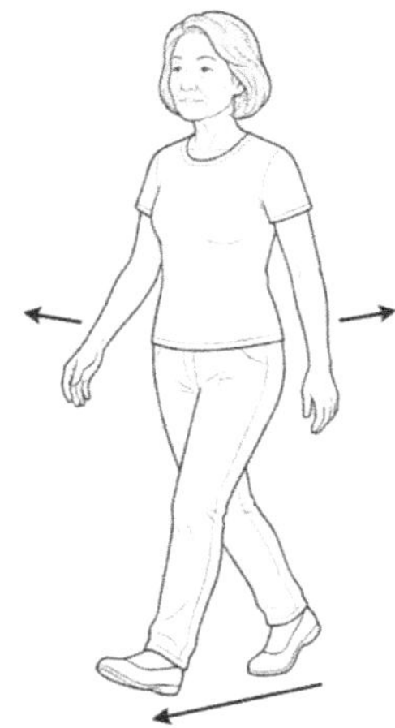

This is not a new movement to master. It is simply the natural arm swing that belongs with the walk. If it feels awkward at first, let it be awkward. After two or three steps it will begin to settle on its own.

- **Reps:** 1–2 passes only in Week 1
- **Rest:** Rooted Stance, 2 breaths between passes
- **When to add:** Day 3 onward; only when the Forward Walk feels steady without it
- **If uncertain:** Return to Movement 3 arms-free for the full session. Add arms the following day.

The Session Close

Every session in this program ends the same way. Not with a final movement, but with three short closing actions that together take less than two minutes and are just as important as anything that came before them.

These three actions are not optional. They are not a cool-down you can skip when you are busy. They are the part of the session where the body settles what it has just learned. Think of them as the period at the end of the sentence. Without them, the session is unfinished.

You will do these in the same order, every session, across all four weeks and beyond.

Close Action 1: Shoulder Rolls

What it is: A slow, deliberate rolling movement of both shoulders, releasing the tension that builds in the upper back and neck during focused balance work.

Why it matters: During balance practice the shoulders quietly tighten. Most people do not notice this happening. The shoulder roll at the close of each session releases that accumulated tension before it settles into stiffness. Seniors who skip this step consistently report more upper back tension the following morning.

How to do it:

1. Stand in the Rooted Stance — feet hip-width apart, knees soft, arms hanging loosely at your sides.
2. Breathe in slowly. As you exhale, lift both shoulders upward toward your ears in a smooth, unhurried shrug.
3. Continue rolling the shoulders backward in a full circle — up, back, down, forward — and let them drop completely at the bottom. Feel the release as they fall. That is two seconds up, two seconds back, two seconds down.

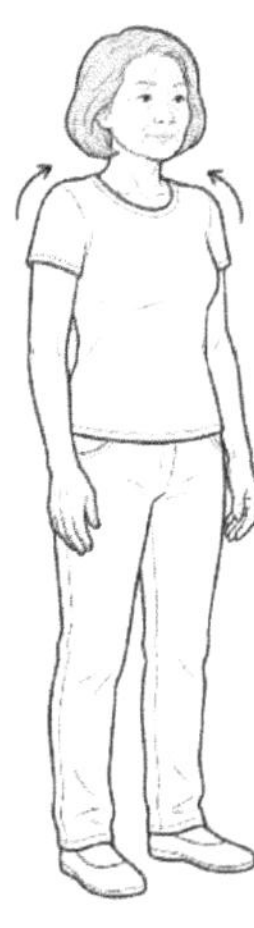

Repeat twice rolling backward. Then twice rolling forward.

Breath cue: Exhale as the shoulders drop. Do not hold the breath.
Reps: × 2 backward, × 2 forward

Close Action 2: Ankle Circles

What it is: Slow circular rotations of each ankle joint, maintaining the mobility that the balance work in this session has just trained.

Why it matters: The ankle is the first joint to receive ground information during walking. The Rooted Stance, the Empty Step, and the Forward Walk all depend on the ankle being mobile, responsive, and well-circulated. Ankle circles at the close of each session keep the joint warm and mobile overnight, so it is ready for the next session without needing extra warm-up time.

How to do it:

1. Stand beside your wall or chair and place one hand lightly on it for support.
2. Shift your weight slightly onto one foot. Lift the other foot just an inch or two off the floor, no higher than needed.
3. Rotate the lifted foot slowly in a full circle at the ankle: forward, out, back, in. Keep the movement smooth and continuous. After 4 full circles in one direction, reverse and rotate 4 circles the other way. Lower the foot. Repeat on the other side.

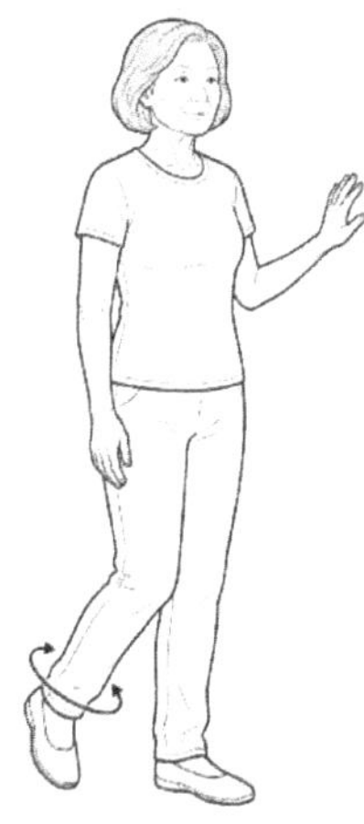

Breath cue: Breathe naturally throughout. Do not hold the breath.
Reps: × 4 circles each direction, each ankle

Close Action 3: The Still Stand

What it is: One full minute of standing quietly in the Rooted Stance after the session is complete.

Why it matters: This is not rest. This is integration. In the sixty seconds after a balance practice session, the nervous system processes and consolidates the motor patterns it has just rehearsed. Research on motor learning consistently shows that a brief period of quiet stillness immediately after practice strengthens the neural encoding of new movement habits more than continuing to move or immediately resuming other activity. The Still Stand is, in functional terms, the most important sixty seconds of the entire session.

How to do it:

1. Return to the Rooted Stance. Feet hip-width apart, knees soft, arms at your sides, crown lifts gently.
2. Close your eyes if that feels comfortable, or soften your gaze toward a fixed point on the floor a few feet ahead.
3. Simply stand. Breathe naturally. Do not perform any movement. Let the body be still. Notice two things: how your feet feel against the floor right now, and whether your breathing feels different from when you began the session. At the end of sixty seconds, open your eyes if closed. You are done.

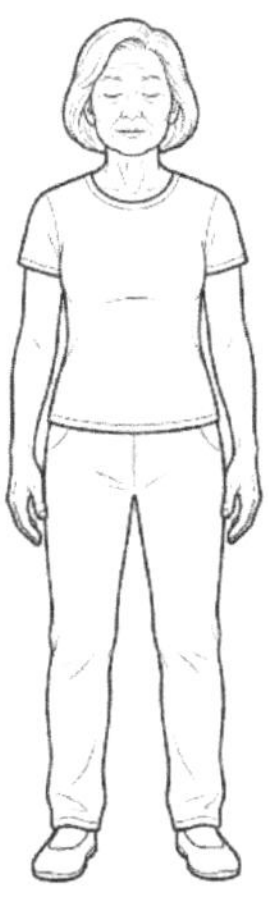

Breath cue: Natural, uncontrolled breath throughout.
Duration: 60 seconds

A Note on the Close for All Four Weeks

The Session Close is identical every session, every week. It does not change as the program progresses. What changes is what you notice during the Still Stand. In Week 1, most people notice only that their feet are tired and their breathing is faster than usual. By Week 4, most people notice that their feet feel more connected to the floor than they did at the start, and that their breathing is slower and calmer at the end of a session than at the beginning. That shift is the practice working.

Week 1 Session Map

Time	Activity
0:00 to 2:00	Arrive — Rooted Stance, three breaths, body scan
2:00 to 3:30	Movement 2 — Empty Step, 4 to 6 cycles
3:30 to 4:00	Rooted Stance reset, two breaths
4:00 to 6:30	Movement 3 — Forward Walk, 3 to 4 passes
6:30 to 8:00	Movement 4 — Forward Walk with Arm Coordination, 1 to 2 passes *(Day 3 onward only)*
8:00 to 8:30	Rooted Stance, shoulder rolls, ankle rotations
8:30 to 10:00	Close — three breaths, noticing

Note: On Days 1 and 2, Movement 4 is not yet added. The time from 6:30 to 8:00 is used as additional Forward Walk practice or extended Rooted Stance rest.

This map is a guide, not a contract. If the Empty Step takes longer on a given day, let it. If you complete fewer passes of the Forward Walk, that is acceptable. The ten minutes is the container. What fills it should respond to how your body is today.

Rest Days

Practice five days and rest two. The rest days are not wasted days. Consolidation of motor learning happens during rest, not during practice. A student who practices seven days a week out of determination will often plateau faster than one who takes their rest days. Trust the structure.

On rest days, a five-minute gentle walk at any pace, outdoors if possible, is beneficial. This is not practice. It is simply keeping the body moving between sessions.

What to Feel For

At the end of each session this week, stand in the Rooted Stance and ask yourself two questions. Not to judge the session, but simply to notice.

Question 1: Did I feel where my weight was during the Empty Step?

Not perfectly, not always, but at least some of the time. Even a momentary sense of the weight being truly on one side and the other foot being genuinely light is significant. That sensation is the beginning of the skill.

Question 2: Did my heel land before the rest of my foot in the Forward Walk?

Again, not every step, but some steps. Some people discover in the first session that they have been landing toe-first for years without realizing it. Noticing this is not failure. It is exactly the kind of awareness this program exists to build.

By Day 5 of this week, most people report that the Empty Step feels slightly more reliable than it did on Day 1. Not dramatically different. Slightly. That is a genuine neurological change. It is enough.

One more thing worth knowing: it is entirely normal to feel more tired after these sessions than the ten-minute duration would seem to justify. Slow, attentive movement is neurologically demanding in a way that brisk, automatic movement is not. Your brain is working hard during these sessions, even when your body is barely moving. A short rest after practice is reasonable and sometimes necessary, particularly in the first week.

Week 2 builds on everything you have practiced here. It will ask you to move in two directions you have not yet trained: sideways and backward. But before that can happen, the weight transfer you are building this week needs to become a little more familiar. That is what Days 1 through 5 are for.

Chapter 7: Week 2 — Steady in All Directions

What Is New This Week

If Week 1 was about slowing down, Week 2 is about expanding.

You spent five sessions learning to shift your weight completely before lifting a foot, and to walk forward with deliberate heel-to-toe contact. That work is not finished, and you will continue it this week. But you are now ready to add two directions that Week 1 deliberately left out: sideways and backward.

This matters for a practical reason that goes beyond the exercise room. Real life does not only move forward. You step sideways to let someone pass in a corridor. You step backward to open a door. You move laterally to reach something on a shelf, to turn in a small bathroom, to navigate a crowded space. The falls that happen in these moments are disproportionately serious because the body has rarely trained for them. A senior with excellent forward balance can still be completely unprepared for the lateral stumble or the unexpected backward step.

Week 2 closes that gap.

The session structure remains identical to Week 1: two minutes to arrive, six to seven minutes of movement, one to two minutes to close. The Rooted Stance and the Empty Step still open and thread through every session. What changes is the movement content of those middle minutes. The Forward Walk continues, and this week it also incorporates the Arm Coordination from Chapter 5. The Side Step and the Backward Step are introduced for the first time.

One student I worked with, a retired postal worker named Gerald who had been avoiding stairs since a near-miss on an escalator, told me at the end of his second week that for the first time in over a year he had stepped sideways to avoid his dog without bracing for disaster. He had not thought about it until afterward. That unawareness, that automatic trust, is exactly what Week 2 is building.

Moving Sideways and Backward

Movement 5: The Side Step

Refer to the full description and illustration in Chapter 5.

This week you will perform the Side Step as a traveling sequence: step right, close, step right, close, for three to four steps in one direction, pause in the Rooted Stance, then reverse and repeat to the left.

- **Repetitions:** 3 to 4 steps each direction, 2 to 3 sets per session
- **Rest:** Rooted Stance with two breaths between each direction change
- **Support:** One hand on the wall beside you until the lateral shift feels reliable
- **Key reminder:** The feet never cross. One steps out, the other closes to hip-width. Always.

The most common error in the Side Step at this stage is the partial weight shift: moving the foot sideways before the weight has fully left it. If the stepping foot feels heavy when it moves, the weight has not fully transferred. Return to the Rooted Stance, reset the weight to the standing foot completely, and try again. There is no penalty for resetting. Resetting is the practice.

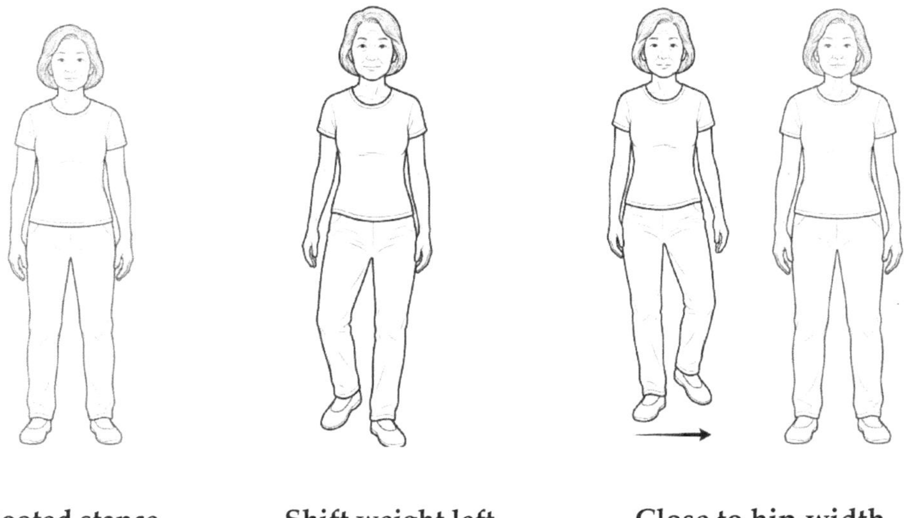

Rooted stance   Shift weight left   Close to hip-width

Movement 6: The Backward Step

Refer to the full description and illustration in Chapter 5.

Perform the Backward Step this week as a short traveling sequence: two steps backward, pause in the Rooted Stance, two steps backward again, for a total of two to three short sequences per session.

- **Repetitions:** 2 backward steps per sequence, 2 to 3 sequences per session
- **Rest:** Rooted Stance with two breaths between each sequence
- **Support:** One hand on the wall beside you for all backward movement this week
- **Safety check:** Before each backward sequence, take a brief glance over one shoulder to confirm the space behind you is clear. Make this a habit from the very first session.
- **Key reminder:** Toes reach back first. The heel lowers after the toes are placed. The spine stays upright. If the upper body is tilting forward to compensate for the backward movement, slow down and reduce the step length.

Backward stepping is one of the movements that surprises students most. Many people discover that their sense of where the floor is behind them is significantly less reliable than their sense of where it is in front. This is normal. It is the result of years of walking almost entirely forward. The proprioceptive pathways for backward movement exist, but they have been underused. Two weeks of consistent backward stepping will noticeably improve this spatial awareness.

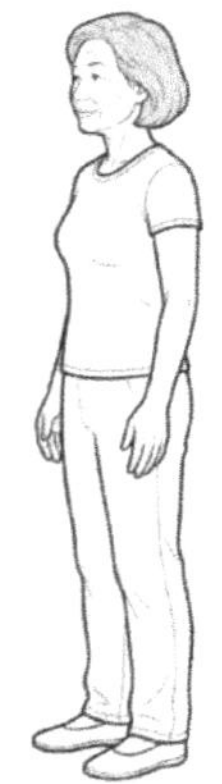

Check space behind

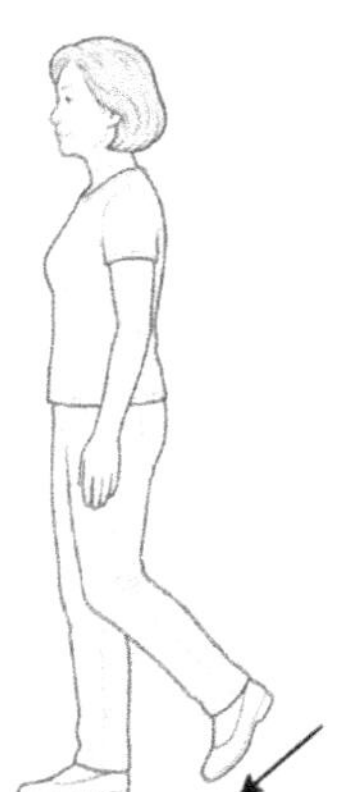

Toes touch first

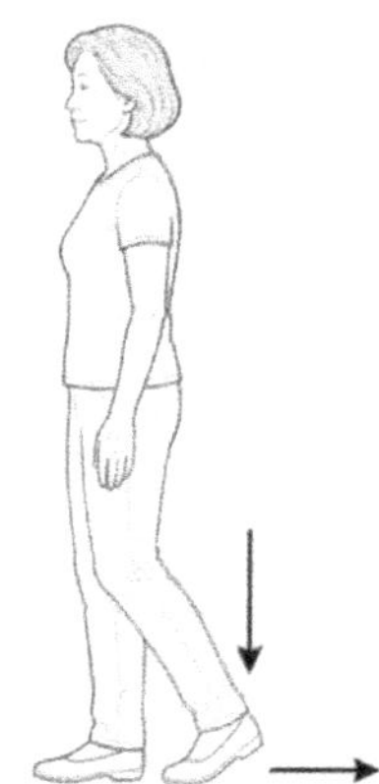

Weight shifts to left foot

The Tai Chi Turn

A note on this movement. The Tai Chi Turn was not included in Chapter 5 with the other core movements, and that was a deliberate choice. A turn only becomes meaningful once there is somewhere to turn from. In the first week you were building the weight transfer and forward walk, and with arm coordination that give the turn its context. Teaching it before Week 1 would have been showing you a door before you had learned how to walk toward it. Now that you have, the Tai Chi Turn is the next natural next step.

Every walking practice, whether in a corridor or a garden path, requires a turn. Most seniors do not think about turns as a balance challenge until they experience a stumble during one. Turns are, in fact, one of the highest-risk moments in walking. The center of mass shifts laterally, the visual field rotates, and the body must reorganize its stability in a fraction of a second.

The Tai Chi Turn addresses this directly. It is not a pivot. It is a series of small, deliberate steps that rotate the body safely and in full control.

Movement 7 — Forward Walk with Arm Coordination and Tai Chi Turn

This is one continuous movement, not three separate ones. The Forward Walk, the Arm Coordination, and the Tai Chi Turn are performed together as a single flowing pass from start to finish.

How to perform it:

Begin in the Rooted Stance. Start the Forward Walk with the heel landing first, rolling through to the toe, full weight transfer before the back foot lifts. As each foot steps forward, the opposite arm swings gently forward; small, relaxed, no higher than the hip. Let this arm swing run naturally through every step of the pass (revisit Week 1's movements for complete illustration).

At the end of the pass, as you prepare to turn, do the following:

1. Come to a full stop in the Rooted Stance. Let the arms settle naturally at the sides.

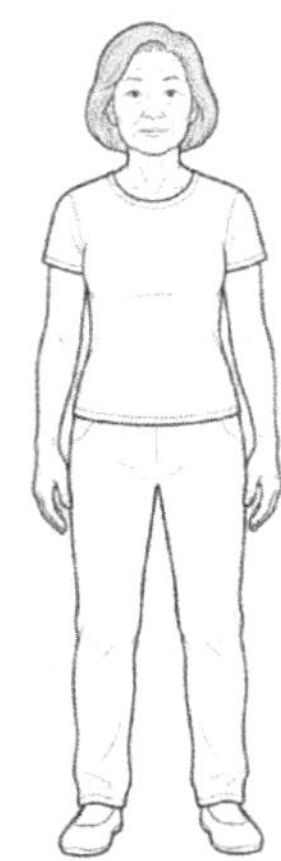

2. Perform the Tai Chi Turn – shift your weight fully to the left foot.

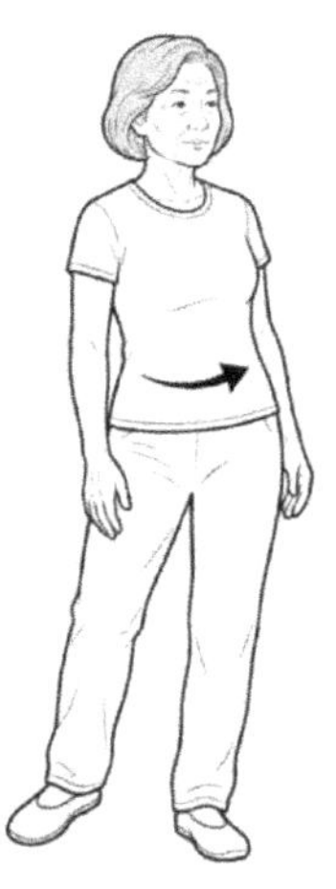

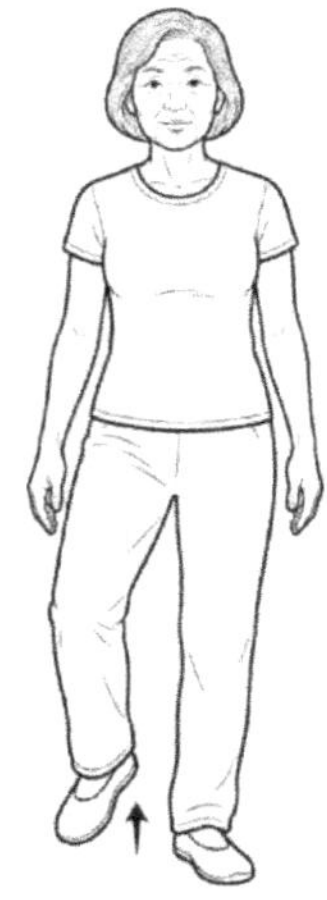

Shift weight left   **Empty right foot**

3. Using small steps, step the right foot out to a slight angle, then shift weight to the right foot.

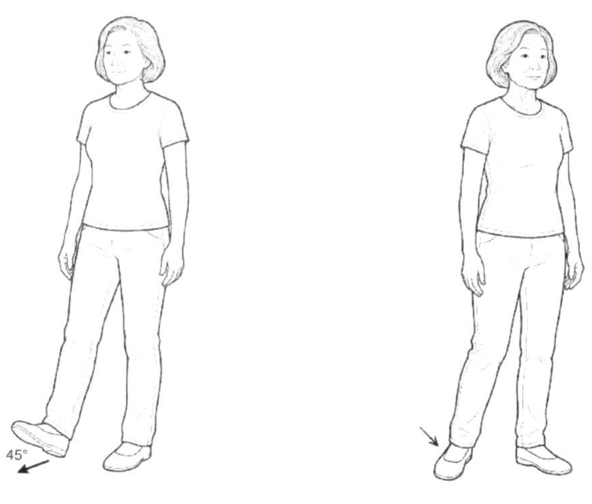

Slight angle   Shift weight right

4. Lift the left foot and bring it around to restore the hip-width stance facing the new direction. You are standing in the Rooted Stance again.

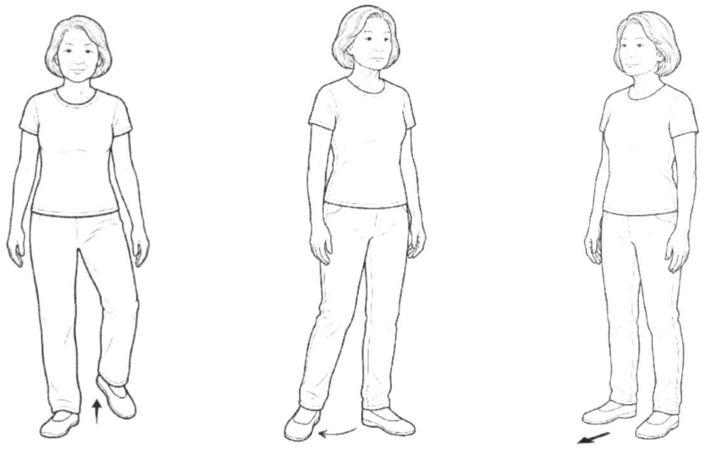

Empty left foot   Rooted stance

5. As soon as the turn is complete and you are back in the Rooted Stance facing the new direction, let the arms resume their natural opposite swing as the Forward Walk begins again

Important note: The arms rest briefly and naturally during the turn itself. They are not swinging during a turn because the body is reorganizing its direction. The moment the new direction is established and the walk resumes, the arm coordination picks up exactly where it left off.

A reminder on the pace of the turn

The full turn takes two to three small steps, never one pivot. At every step, the full Empty Step rule applies that has applied since Week 1: weight travels completely before any foot lifts. When in doubt, slow down.

Keep the gaze forward throughout the turn. Do not look down at the feet. The eyes looking forward helps the vestibular system maintain orientation during the rotation.

- **Repetitions:** 2 full passes; Use the Tai Chi Turn at the end of every Forward Walk with arm coordination.

  Note: A pass is one complete walk from one end of your practice space to the other end; and the reverse counts as a second pass and so on.

- **Rest:** Rooted Stance, 2 breaths between passes

  E.g. Walk forward with arm coordination to the end of your practice space. Do a Tai Chi Turn. Walk back with arm coordination. Do another Tai Chi Turn. That is one pass. Rest 2 breaths in Rooted Stance. Repeat for a second pass.

- **Support:** Fingertips on the wall during the turn if the rotation feels uncertain. Wall contact during the turn until it feels reliable
- **Key reminder:** Small steps. Never a pivot on one foot. Weight transfers at every step of the turn.

Week 2 Session Map

The session structure is identical to Week 1. The movement content changes as follows:

Time	Activity
0:00 to 2:00	Arrive — Rooted Stance, three breaths, body scan
2:00 to 3:00	Movement 2 — Empty Step, 4 to 6 cycles

Time	Activity
3:00 to 4:30	Movement 7 — Forward Walk with Arm Coordination and Tai Chi Turn. Walk to end, turn, walk back, turn — twice
4:30 to 5:00	Rooted Stance reset, two breaths
5:00 to 6:30	Movement 5 — Side Step, 3 to 4 steps each direction, 2 sets
6:30 to 7:30	Movement 6 — Backward Step, 2 steps per sequence, 2 sequences
7:30 to 8:30	Rooted Stance, shoulder rolls, ankle rotations
8:30 to 10:00	Close — three breaths, noticing

If this feels like a lot in the first session of Week 2, reduce the Side Step and Backward Step to one set each. The aim is to touch each movement every session, not to exhaust yourself completing a fixed quota.

What to Feel For

At the end of each session this week, bring the same two-question check-in from Week 1, and add a third.

Question 1: Did the weight shift feel more complete than it did in Week 1?

Even slightly. Even occasionally. Any movement in this direction is real.

Question 2: Did the heel land first in the Forward Walk, more consistently than last week?

Question 3: Did I feel uncertain during the Side Step or Backward Step, and did I stay with it anyway?

That third question matters because the feeling of uncertainty during a new movement is not a sign that something is wrong. It is the sign that the nervous system is genuinely working. Comfortable movements do not build balance. Movements that are slightly outside the familiar range, performed slowly and with support, do.

By Day 5 of this week, the Side Step should feel less unfamiliar. The Backward Step may still feel tentative, and that is normal. The Tai Chi Turn will have replaced the informal shuffle you used to change direction in Week 1, and it may already feel noticeably more organized.

Week 3 asks the body for something new: coordination between the upper and lower body, and a step that asks the knee to lift with intention rather than simply clear the floor. The foundation you are building this week makes that possible. Keep showing up.

Chapter 8: Week 3 — Coordination and Quiet Strength

What Your Body Has Been Building

Something has been happening in your body across the past two weeks that you may not yet have fully noticed.

The stabilizing muscles of the hips and ankles have been working in ways they have not been asked to work in a long time, possibly years. The proprioceptive pathways in the soles of your feet have been receiving deliberate, repeated stimulation. The vestibular system has been processing the slow, controlled postural shifts of the Empty Step hundreds of times. The nervous system has been building and refining new motor patterns through consistent, attentive repetition.

None of this is dramatic. None of it announces itself. But it is real, and Week 3 is where it begins to become visible.

Most of my students notice the change first not during practice, but during ordinary daily movement. They reach for something on a shelf and realize they did it without bracing. They step over a threshold and notice they did not hesitate. A student named Dorothy, who had been gripping stair railings with both hands since a fall two years before, told me at the start of her third week that she had gone down the stairs using only one hand and had not thought anything of it until she was already at the bottom. She stood at the foot of the stairs for a moment, she said, just slightly amazed.

That is the change this program builds. Not dramatic displays of athletic ability. The recovery of ordinary ease.

Week 3 introduces two new movements: Cloud Hands Walking, which trains upper and lower body coordination through a flowing arm movement, and the Tandem Walk, which challenges narrow-base balance in a controlled, supported context. Both movements build on the weight transfer skills you have developed in Weeks 1 and 2. Neither can be performed well without them.

A word before you begin this movement: Cloud Hands Walking and the Tandem Walk that follows it were not introduced in Chapter 5. They were held back deliberately. Both movements depend on the weight transfer precision and postural control you have been building for two weeks. Introduced before that foundation existed, they would have been difficult, discouraging, and possibly unsafe. Introduced now, they are exactly what the body is ready for. This is not a program that withholds for the sake of it. It is a program that sequences for a reason. You will find that both movements, challenging as they may feel on Day 1, become noticeably more natural across the five sessions of this week.

The week also continues all the movements from Weeks 1 and 2. The Empty Step, the Forward Walk with Arm Coordination, the Side Step, the Backward Step, and the Tai Chi Turn all remain in the session. The new movements are added alongside them, not instead of them. This cumulative approach is not about making the session harder. It is about building a complete movement vocabulary that covers all the directions and coordination patterns a senior might need in daily life.

Cloud Hands Walking

Movement 8: Cloud Hands Walking

Cloud Hands is one of the most recognizable movements in Tai Chi. In its full form it is a flowing, continuous arm-and-torso rotation performed while stepping sideways. In this program, it is adapted into a walking version that can be performed moving forward and that trains something no previous movement in this program has addressed directly: coordinated rotation between the upper and lower body.

When the arms and torso rotate with the legs in a coordinated pattern during walking, the spine becomes an active stabilizer rather than a passive passenger. The deep rotational muscles of the trunk, the obliques and the multifidus, engage continuously throughout the movement. These are the muscles responsible for protecting the spine during twisting, for maintaining upright posture during asymmetric loads, and for contributing to the smooth transfer of force from the lower body to the upper body in every step.

How to perform Cloud Hands Walking:

1. Begin in the Rooted Stance. Take a slow breath to settle.
2. As you begin to step forward with the right foot, raise the right arm in a gentle arc, palm facing inward, until the hand reaches approximately shoulder height in front of you. At the same time, lower the left arm in a mirror arc, palm facing outward and downward, until it rests near the left hip.

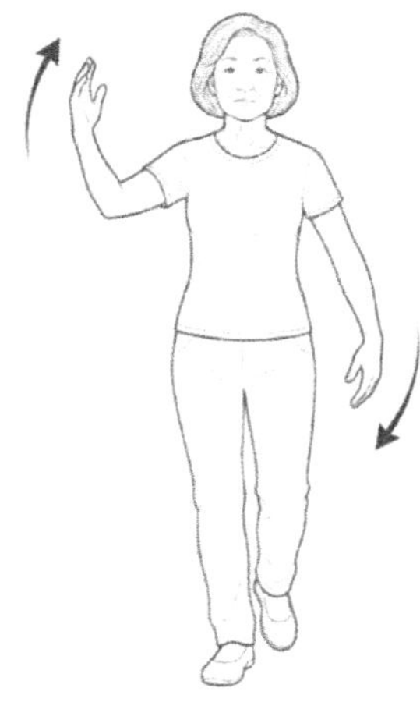

3. As your weight transfers to the right foot and the left foot steps forward, the arms exchange positions: the left arm rises in the same gentle arc while the right descends.

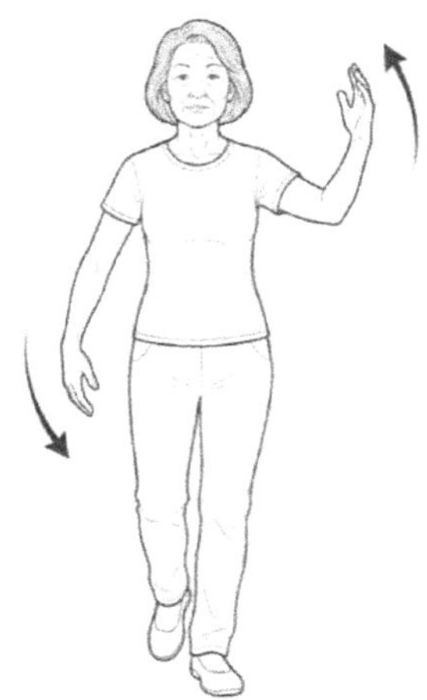

The movement is slow, smooth, and continuous, like water flowing in two direction simultaneously.

The upper body does not twist aggressively. The rotation is gentle and comes from the relaxation of the torso rather than from muscular effort. Think of the arms as the visible expression of the internal rotation, not the cause of it.

- **Repetitions:** 4 to 6 steps per pass, 2 to 3 passes per session
- **Rest:** Rooted Stance with two breaths between passes
- **Support:** Reduce the arm height initially if raising one arm to shoulder height disturbs balance. Hands at mid-torso height are perfectly acceptable and produce the same rotational benefit.
- **Key reminder:** Arm and step move together. The arm should not be leading or trailing the step. They coordinate as one.

The Higher Step and Tandem Walk

Movement 9: The Controlled High Step

A word before you begin this movement: You did not see this movement in Chapter 5. That was intentional. The Controlled High Step requires a standing leg that can hold full body weight with confidence while the opposite knee lifts and holds. That confidence takes time to build. The two weeks behind you have been building it. You are ready for this now in a way you were not on Day 1.

The Controlled High Step introduces a gentle deliberate knee lift during the Forward Walk. It is not a marching step. The knee lifts only to a comfortable height, typically to a point where the thigh is parallel with the floor or lower, and the movement is slow and fully controlled throughout.

This also matters because the hip flexor engagement and single-leg balance time required by a higher knee lift are significantly greater than in a normal walking step. Stairs, curbs, and uneven terrain all require the body to lift the foot higher than flat-floor walking demands. Seniors who have not practiced this movement regularly often find their toe clearance when stepping up a curb is minimal, which is one of the most common causes of trip-and-fall injuries.

How to perform it:

1. From the Rooted Stance, shift weight fully to the left foot using the Empty Step.

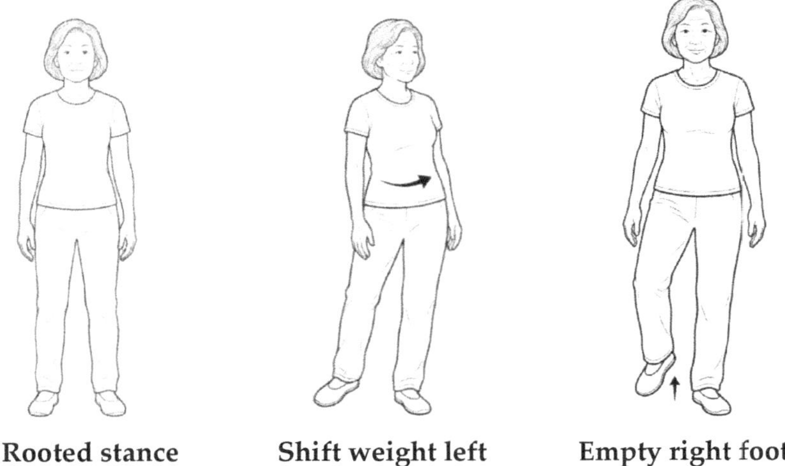

2. Slowly lift the right knee until it reaches a comfortable height, pause briefly at the top of the lift with the right foot hanging relaxed

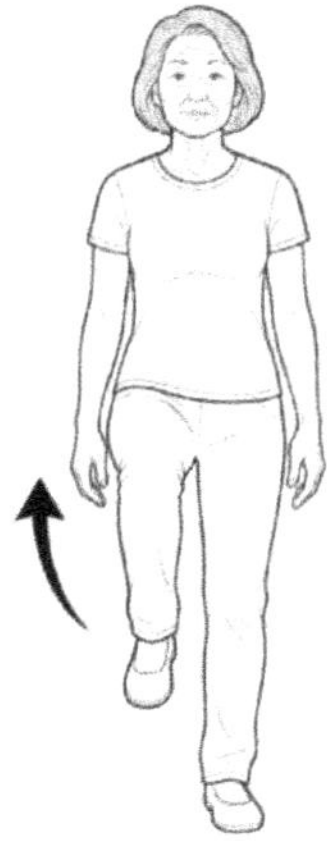

3. Then lower the right foot forward to the floor with heel-first contact, as in the Forward Walk.

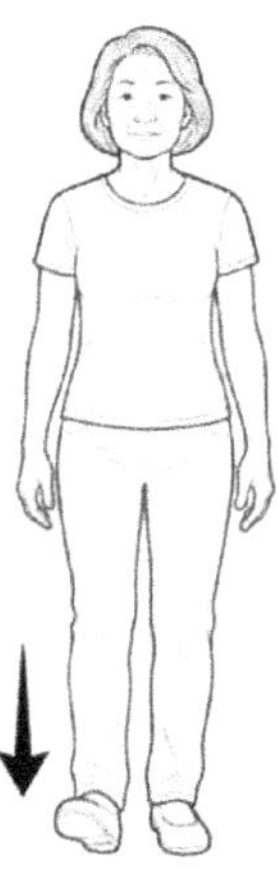

4. Repeat with the left leg. Move slowly throughout.

- **Repetitions:** 4 to 6 steps per pass, 2 passes per session
- **Rest:** Rooted Stance between passes
- **Support:** One hand on wall or chair back throughout this movement until single-leg balance during the knee lift feels stable
- **Key reminder:** The standing leg does the work. The lifting leg is relaxed. Do not tense the lifting foot. Let it hang.

Movement 10: The Tandem Walk

The Tandem Walk places one foot directly in front of the other along a straight line, heel of the front foot touching or nearly touching the toes of the back foot.

This narrow-base stance challenges balance more directly than the hip-width stance of the Forward Walk and brings the body's balance systems into focused engagement.

This is not a test of perfection. It is a practice. If the feet cannot land directly in line, a near-line is sufficient. The value is in the narrow base, not in achieving a geometrically precise straight line.

How to perform it:

1. Stand at the wall with one hand available for support. Take a slow breath.

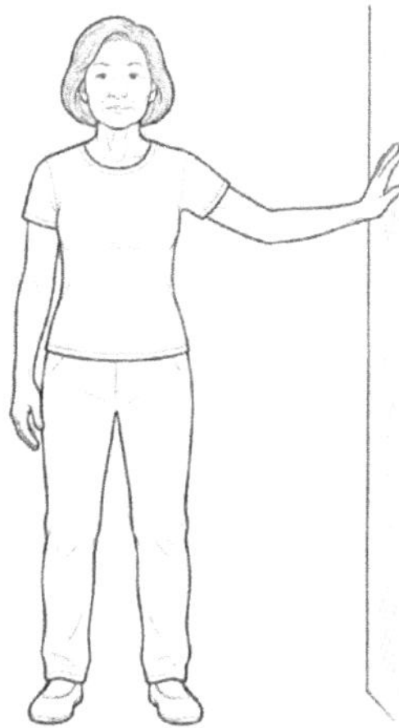

2. Step the right foot forward and place it directly in front of the left foot, heel-close to or touching the left toes. Shift weight to the right foot.

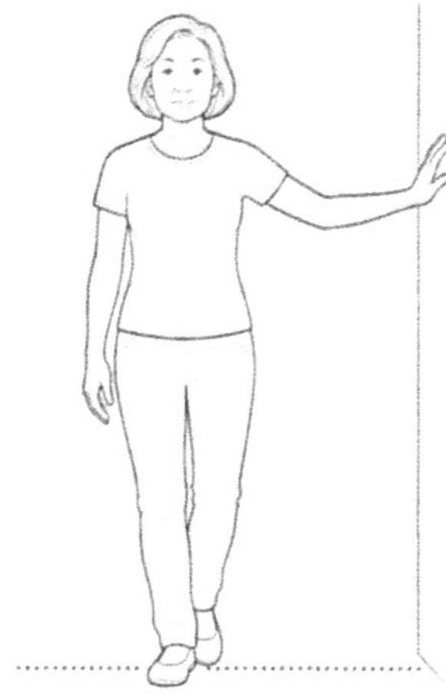

3. Step the left foot forward and place it in front of the right in the same way.

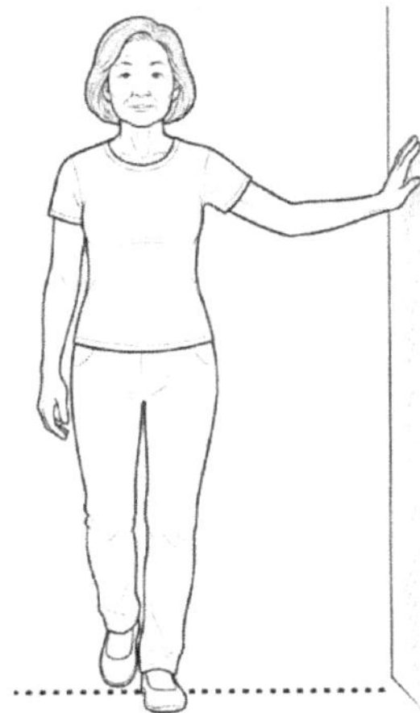

Continue for four to six steps, maintaining the narrow line. Keep the gaze forward and the spine upright throughout.

- **Repetitions:** 4 to 6 steps per pass, 2 passes per session
- **Rest:** Full return to hip-width Rooted Stance between passes
- **Support:** Fingertips on wall throughout. This is not a movement to practice without a wall nearby in Week 3.
- **Key reminder:** If the body sways significantly during the Tandem Walk, widen the line slightly. A slightly wider narrow base still provides most of the training benefit with reduced risk.

Week 3 Session Map

Time	Activity
0:00 to 2:00	Arrive — Rooted Stance, three breaths, body scan
2:00 to 3:00	Movement 2 — Empty Step, 4 to 6 cycles
3:00 to 4:00	Movement 7 — Forward Walk with Arm Coordination and Tai Chi Turn, walk to end, turn, walk back, turn — twice
4:00 to 5:00	Movement 8 — Cloud Hands Walking, 4 to 6 steps, 2 to 3 passes

Time	Activity
5:00 to 5:30	Rooted Stance reset, two breaths
5:30 to 6:30	Movement 9 — Controlled High Step, 4 to 6 steps, 2 passes
6:30 to 7:30	Movement 10 — Tandem Walk, 4 to 6 steps, 2 passes with wall support
7:30 to 8:30	Movements 5 and 6 — Side Step and Backward Step, 1 set each as review
8:30 to 10:00	Close — Rooted Stance, shoulder rolls, ankle circles, three breaths, noticing

If this session feels full, drop the Side Step and Backward Step review in the final minutes and extend the closing rest instead. The new movements, Cloud Hands Walking, the Controlled High Step, and the Tandem Walk, are the priority this week.

What to Feel For

Week 3 introduces a new quality of self-check. In addition to the questions from Weeks 1 and 2, ask:

Question 1: Did the arms and legs feel connected during Cloud Hands Walking, even briefly?

Even one moment of genuine coordination, one step where the arm and leg moved as one thing, is significant. That is the motor pattern being established.

Question 2: Did the standing leg feel solid during the Controlled High Step?

Not perfectly still. Solid. There is a difference. A wobble with a firm base is different from a wobble with an uncertain one.

Question 3: Did the Tandem Walk feel less precarious by Day 5 than it did on Day 1?

Most people find that it does. The improvement across five sessions of the Tandem Walk is often one of the most noticeable changes seniors experience in the entire four-week program. The narrow base forces the balance system to adapt quickly, and it does.

Dorothy, whose staircase story opened this chapter, completed Week 3 and told me afterward that the Tandem Walk had been the movement she was most uncertain about. By Day 4 she was completing four steps without touching the wall. That was not the goal. It was simply what happened when she showed up and let the body do its work.

Week 4 takes everything built across the three weeks and allows it to become a single flowing practice. You will not be adding new individual movements. You will be putting everything together, and then you will be taking it outside.

Chapter 9: Week 4 — The Full Practice

What Week 4 Is

Week 4 is not harder than Week 3. It is deeper.

No new movements are introduced this week. Every movement you need is already in your body, built over fifteen sessions across three weeks of consistent practice. What Week 4 asks is something different: that you let those movements connect into a single, flowing practice rather than a sequence of separate exercises performed one at a time.

In the first three weeks, the session map was a structure to hold onto. A sequence of discrete movements with clear boundaries between them. That structure served its purpose. It gave the nervous system clear, separable tasks to learn. It prevented overwhelm. It allowed each skill to develop without competition from the others.

Week 4 dissolves those boundaries, gently. The movements no longer stop and start in separate slots. They flow from one to the next with the Rooted Stance as a breath between them rather than a wall between them. The Empty Step is no longer an isolated exercise at the top of the session. It is embedded in every step you take. The Tai Chi Turn connects the Forward Walk with arm coordination to the Side Step. The Cloud Hands Walking leads naturally into the Controlled High Step. The session begins to feel less like a series of tasks and more like a practice.

This is what Tai Chi Walking is meant to feel like. And for most of my students, it is in Week 4 that they first experience it that way.

The Week 4 Flowing Session

Rather than a time-slotted map, this week uses a flowing sequence. Move through each element at your own pace, using the Rooted Stance with a single breath as the transition between elements. If you lose the thread of the sequence, return to the Rooted Stance, take one breath, and continue from wherever you are.

Flowing Sequence:

1. Arrive in the Rooted Stance

Three slow breaths. Full body scan from feet to crown. Notice one thing about how your body feels today. Do not judge it. Simply note it.

2. Empty Step

Six cycles, alternating sides, moving slightly more slowly than feels necessary. Let this be a deliberate arrival in the body, not a warm-up to get through.

3. Forward Walk with Arm Coordination

Four passes with the Tai Chi Turn at each end. Let the breath coordinate naturally. On the third and fourth pass, introduce the Cloud Hands arm movement in place of the standard Arm Coordination. Allow the transition between the two arm styles to happen as a gradual drift rather than a sudden change.

4. Controlled High Step

Woven into the Forward Walk rather than performed as a separate sequence. On the third or fourth step of each pass, allow one step to become a High Step, with the knee lifting with intention before the heel lands. Then return to the ordinary Forward Walk pace. Do not flag or announce it. Simply let it appear and disappear within the walking.

5. Side Steps

Four steps in each direction, two sets. These follow naturally after the Forward Walk passes. Think of them not as a different exercise but as a change of direction within the same practice.

6. Backward Steps

Two steps backward, pause, two more. Three sequences. After the final sequence, the Tai Chi Turn brings you back to the forward-facing direction and directly into the next element.

7. Tandem Walk

Four to six steps, two passes, wall within reach. By Day 3 or 4 of this week, try the first pass without touching the wall unless needed. The wall remains nearby. The fingertips simply lift away from it.

8. Close

Return to the Rooted Stance. Three slow breaths. Shoulder rolls. Ankle circles. Stand still for sixty seconds and notice two things: how your feet feel against the floor, and whether your breathing is different from when you began.

The full sequence should take ten minutes at the pace this program has established. If it regularly takes eleven or twelve, that is not a problem. If it consistently takes under eight, you are moving too quickly.

Taking the Practice Outside

From Day 3 of this week onward, one of your five practice days can take place outdoors.

This is a meaningful transition. The indoor practice environment of the past three weeks has been controlled, predictable, and familiar. The floor is level, the light is consistent, and there are no competing sensory demands. This control was deliberate. It gave the nervous system the clearest possible conditions in which to learn the new movement patterns.

Outdoors, everything changes slightly. The surface is uneven in ways no indoor floor is. The light shifts. There is wind. There are other people, sounds, and visual distractions. The feet receive different feedback through the soles. The vestibular system has more to process. The dual-task demand, moving while also navigating an environment, is higher.

This is not a reason to avoid outdoor practice. It is the reason outdoor practice is so valuable. The real world is where the balance this program builds will be used. Bringing the practice into that environment, under controlled conditions, is the final step in transferring what has been learned from the indoor training session to daily life.

Guidelines for outdoor practice:

Choose a flat, quiet surface for the first outdoor session. A paved path in a park, a quiet stretch of pavement, or a flat area of garden are all suitable. Avoid wet surfaces, loose gravel, and any area with significant foot traffic on the first day.

Wear the same appropriate flat-soled footwear used indoors. This is not the day for sandals or unfamiliar shoes.

Begin with the Rooted Stance as always. Take an extra breath here and notice the outdoor environment with all your senses before you begin to move. Let the sounds, the air, the light, and the ground beneath you simply register. You are not ignoring them. You are acknowledging them and then allowing your attention to settle inward to the practice.

Perform the full flowing sequence. Move at the same pace as indoors. The outdoor environment will naturally create small additional challenges. Allow them. Do not attempt to eliminate the variability. The variability is the training.

If the surface becomes uneven mid-practice, pause in the Rooted Stance, assess the ground ahead, and either continue slowly or step to a more level area. There is no benefit in pressing through unsafe terrain. The body learns balance from manageable challenge, not from situations that exceed its current capacity.

What most people discover:

Within two or three outdoor sessions, most seniors find that walking outdoors begins to feel noticeably different from how it felt before the program. Not always dramatically. Often in small ways. The foot notices the slight slope of a pavement. The body adjusts without being asked to consciously. A step onto a grass verge that might previously have produced a moment of anxiety instead produces only a slight, automatic adjustment and nothing more.

That is transfer. That is the practice working in the world. That is what Week 4 is for.

A Note on Consistency Beyond Week 4

This program ends at the close of Week 4. The practice does not.

The movements you have built across these four weeks are not a course you complete. They are a practice you continue. The research is clear on this: balance improvements achieved through Tai Chi practice diminish over time if the practice stops, and are maintained or continue to improve if the practice continues. Ten minutes a day, five days a week, is all that is needed to maintain and build on what you have established here.

The Bonus 10-Minute Daily Practice Companion at the back of this book gives you a week-by-week visual guide designed to sit flat beside you during sessions so you never need to search for a page while you are moving. It includes the full sequence of all eight movements condensed into a single reference page for each week of ongoing practice.

Many seniors find that after four weeks, ten minutes is no longer a discipline. It is simply a part of the morning, as natural and unremarkable as a cup of tea. When that happens, the practice has found its place.

The Week 4 Self-Check

At the close of the final session of this week, stand in the Rooted Stance for one full minute. Let the breath settle. Then ask yourself these questions, not for evaluation, but for awareness.

Does this feel different from Week 1 Day 1?

Most seniors answer yes to this without hesitation. The body knows. The feet know. The legs know. The simple act of standing in the Rooted Stance in Week 4 carries a quality of settledness that was not there on Day 1, because the nervous system that produces it has been changed by the practice.

Is there a moment in daily life this week that felt different from before the program?

It does not have to be large. Margaret noticed the stairs. Gerald noticed the sideways step around his dog. Dorothy noticed the staircase rail she no longer gripped with both hands. For some people it is a reaching movement, or a moment of turning quickly to respond to someone calling their name, or simply the absence of the brief internal brace that used to precede every step on an uneven surface.

These moments are the point. They are not side effects of the practice. They are the practice, expressed in the world.

Chapter 10: Movement with Your Specific Conditions

How to Use This Chapter

This chapter is for seniors who are managing one or more health conditions that affect movement, balance, or pain levels during physical activity. It covers five of the most common conditions encountered in this practice: arthritis, osteoporosis, Parkinson's disease, peripheral neuropathy, and walking with an assistive device such as a cane or walker.

If none of these apply to you, this chapter is still worth reading once. Understanding how the program adapts to different bodies deepens your understanding of the movements themselves, and you may find information here that is relevant to someone you know.

If one or more of these conditions do apply to you, read the relevant section before you begin Week 1 and carry those modifications into every session from the start. You do not need to wait until a difficulty arises to apply a modification. Building it in from the beginning is always preferable to adjusting under pressure.

A note that applies across all conditions in this chapter: the modifications described here are not lesser versions of the program. They are the program, adapted for the body that is here today. The training principles, the weight transfer, the attentive slowness, the breath coordination, and the consistent daily repetition, remain identical. Only the expression changes.

Arthritis

Arthritis is the most common health condition among seniors and one of the most variable. Two people with osteoarthritis of the knee can have experiences that are almost nothing alike, one managing mild morning stiffness that eases within an hour, the other navigating significant daily pain and limited range of motion. The modifications below apply most directly to arthritis affecting the hips, knees, ankles, and feet, since these are the joints most involved in the movements of this program.

The fundamental principle for arthritis: Move within your pain-free range on every session day, and never push into pain. Mild discomfort during movement, the feeling of joint stiffness being asked to shift, is different from pain. Pain is a signal to reduce the range of motion, slow down further, or stop and rest. Stiffness that eases after two or three minutes of gentle movement is normal for most arthritic joints and is not a reason to avoid practice.

Morning stiffness: Many seniors with arthritis find that the joints are at their stiffest in the first hour after waking. If this applies to you, scheduling practice for mid-morning rather than immediately after rising will allow the joints to warm up naturally before the session begins. A ten-minute gentle walk before the session, even just around the house, can serve the same purpose.

The Rooted Stance: If standing with knees soft causes knee pain, reduce the bend to the smallest degree of softness that is comfortable. Locked knees are not the goal, but forced bent knees are not necessary either. The optimal knee position for arthritic joints is the least bent position that still allows full muscular engagement.

The Empty Step: If full weight transfer to one side produces hip or knee pain on the standing side, reduce the degree of transfer. A ninety percent weight shift is still highly effective training. The foot does not need to be completely weightless to benefit from the practice. Over time, as the stabilizing muscles strengthen, the standing joint will be better supported and the full weight shift will become more comfortable.

The Forward Walk: Reduce the stride length if hip flexion or extension produces pain. A shorter, more deliberate step that is pain-free is more beneficial than a longer step performed with compensatory tension.

The Controlled High Step: If knee flexion beyond a comfortable range produces pain during the knee lift, simply lift the foot to whatever height is comfortable. Even a two-inch lift provides meaningful hip flexor and single-leg balance training. The height of the lift is not the point. The controlled deliberateness of the lift is the point.

The Tandem Walk: If hip or knee pain makes the narrow base of the Tandem Walk uncomfortable, widen the line by two to three inches. This reduces the balance challenge slightly but eliminates the compensatory tension that unmanaged pain creates, which is far more disruptive to balance training than a slightly wider base.

General guidance: Warm the joints before practice with gentle seated ankle circles and knee lifts in a chair if needed. After practice, allow the joints to rest for a few minutes before resuming normal activity. Ice on particularly reactive joints after a session is appropriate if it is part of your usual arthritis management.

Osteoporosis

Osteoporosis reduces bone density and increases the risk of fracture from falls, but it does not prevent physical activity. In fact, weight-bearing exercise is one of the most consistently recommended interventions for maintaining bone density and reducing fracture risk in seniors with osteoporosis. The movements in this program are low-impact and weight-bearing, which is precisely the combination recommended in clinical guidelines.

The modifications for osteoporosis are primarily about avoiding high-risk positions rather than reducing activity.

Avoid spinal flexion: Deep forward bending, particularly under load, increases the risk of vertebral compression fractures in bones with reduced density. None of the movements in this program require deep forward bending. If you find yourself hunching forward during the Forward Walk or the Cloud Hands Walking, consciously return to the upright spinal position described in the Rooted Stance. This is both a safety consideration and a quality of practice consideration.

The Tandem Walk: Walk with particular attention to having the wall within fingertip reach throughout this movement. A fall during the Tandem Walk from a narrow-base stumble carries more consequence for a person with osteoporosis than for someone without. The movement is still appropriate and valuable. The wall contact is non-negotiable.

The Backward Step: Perform with one hand on the wall throughout the entire program, not just in Week 2. The risk of losing balance in the backward direction and falling onto the hip or spine is higher in the context of osteoporosis, and the wall provides reliable protection.

The Controlled High Step: Perform with wall support for the full four weeks. The single-leg balance demand of the knee lift is significant, and the wall ensures that any momentary loss of balance is caught before it becomes a fall.

General guidance: If you have had a vertebral fracture or have been diagnosed with severe osteoporosis, discuss the program specifically with your healthcare provider before beginning, and share this book with them if possible. Most will approve the program with the modifications above already built in.

Parkinson's Disease

Parkinson's disease affects movement in ways that make Tai Chi Walking particularly relevant and particularly valuable. The hallmark movement challenges of Parkinson's, including freezing of gait, reduced stride length, stooped posture, reduced arm swing, and difficulty initiating movement, are addressed directly by the core mechanics of this practice.

Research on Tai Chi for Parkinson's disease is robust. A landmark randomized controlled trial published in the New England Journal of Medicine in 2012 found that Tai Chi training in people with Parkinson's produced significant improvements in balance, stride length, and reduced fall rates compared to both resistance training and stretching. These improvements persisted at a three-month follow-up after the intervention ended.

Freezing of gait: Freezing, the sudden inability to initiate or continue movement during walking, is one of the most disabling and frightening symptoms of Parkinson's. The slow, highly structured movement of Tai Chi Walking provides a natural countermeasure. The attention-based nature of the practice keeps the prefrontal cortex engaged in movement initiation throughout each session, which research suggests partially compensates for the basal ganglia dysfunction responsible for freezing.

If freezing occurs during practice, do not try to push through it or force the step. Instead, perform the following: shift your attention to your breathing, take one long slow exhale, then look at a fixed point on the floor slightly ahead of your feet and step toward it. This cognitive redirect, using visual targeting to initiate movement, is one of the most well-supported strategies for resolving a freeze and is entirely compatible with the principles of this practice.

Arm swing: Parkinson's characteristically reduces arm swing, particularly on the affected side. The Arm Coordination and Cloud Hands Walking movements in this program directly address this. Consciously initiating the arm swing at the start of each Forward Walk pass, even if it feels exaggerated or mechanical, gradually re-establishes the habit of coordinated arm movement. Do not wait for the arm swing to feel natural before doing it. Do it, and the naturalness will develop through repetition.

Posture: The forward-flexed posture common in Parkinson's is directly countered by the upright spine instruction of the Rooted Stance. In every session, return attention to the crown-of-the-head lift and the tailbone-dropping-downward image from Chapter 5 as frequently as needed. Many people with Parkinson's find that this postural attention during practice gradually carries over into their everyday movement.

Session timing: Parkinson's symptoms vary significantly across the day, particularly in relation to medication timing. Schedule practice sessions during the period when your medication is most effective and your movement is most fluid. This maximizes the quality of the motor learning in each session.

Support: Use wall or chair support for all movements throughout the program. There is no timeline for reducing support in the context of Parkinson's. The goal is consistent, safe, daily practice, not independence from support.

Peripheral Neuropathy

Peripheral neuropathy reduces or distorts sensation in the feet and lower legs, which directly impairs the proprioceptive system described in Chapter 1. Seniors with neuropathy often describe their feet as feeling numb, tingly, burning, or as though they are walking on cotton wool. The ground feedback that most people take for granted is simply not arriving clearly.

This makes every element of this program relevant. The deliberate foot-to-floor attention embedded in every movement, particularly the heel-first landing of the Forward Walk and the four-corner contact focus of the Rooted Stance, compensates for reduced proprioception by bringing conscious attention to what the automatic system can no longer provide reliably.

Compensate with vision: In the early weeks of practice, use visual confirmation of foot placement more actively than the standard instruction to keep the gaze forward would suggest. Glancing down at the foot as it lands to confirm placement is acceptable and sensible for neuropathy. As confidence builds, gradually reduce the frequency of these glances and increase the reliance on the available proprioceptive sensation, however limited.

Footwear: Choose footwear that provides the firmest possible ground connection without being thin to the point of providing no protection. Some seniors with neuropathy find that slightly textured insoles enhance what ground sensation remains. This is worth experimenting with.

The Empty Step: This movement is particularly important for neuropathy. Because the reduced sensation makes it harder to feel whether the foot is weighted or not, practice the weight shift slowly and use visual observation of your own body to confirm what sensation cannot. Watch the standing leg press into the floor. Watch the lifting foot come free of the ground. These visual confirmations replace and reinforce the proprioceptive information that sensation would normally provide.

Pacing: Neuropathy can cause foot fatigue and discomfort after sustained standing. If ten minutes becomes uncomfortable before the session ends, reduce the session to eight minutes and build back to ten over the first two weeks. The consistency of daily practice matters more than the exact duration of each session.

Walking with an Assistive Device

Many seniors use a cane, walking stick, or wheeled walker as part of their daily mobility. This program is fully compatible with assistive device use and does not require you to practice without your device if doing so would feel unsafe.

Cane use: Most of the movements in this program can be performed with a cane in the hand opposite the weaker side, as in standard cane use. The Empty Step can be performed with the cane tip lightly on the floor for balance reassurance rather than weight bearing. The Forward Walk can incorporate the cane in its usual position, touching down with the opposite foot as normal cane gait prescribes. The Side Step and Backward Step are performed with the cane available in the usual hand. The Tandem Walk can be performed with the cane touching the floor or the wall providing additional support.

The Arm Coordination and Cloud Hands Walking will naturally be adapted to one-arm movement, with the cane-holding arm remaining relatively stable while the free arm performs the arc movement. This asymmetric version still produces meaningful rotational training through the torso.

Walker use: A standard wheeled walker can be used for the Rooted Stance, the Empty Step, and the Forward Walk, with both hands on the walker frame. The Side Step can be performed with the walker repositioned to the side as each step proceeds. The Backward Step with a walker requires care: move the walker back first, then step back to meet it, one step at a time. The Tandem Walk and the Controlled High Step are best performed with one hand on the wall rather than the walker, as the walker's width makes narrow-base placement difficult.

If you use a rollator walker with brakes, ensure the brakes are engaged during any stationary balance work such as the Empty Step and the Rooted Stance.

The goal: The goal of this program for assistive device users is not to practice without the device. It is to build the balance strength and movement quality that makes the device easier and more confident to use, and that reduces reliance on it where that is safely possible over time. Some seniors do find that their assistive device becomes less necessary after several weeks of consistent practice. Others do not. Both outcomes are valid. The practice serves the body as it is.

A Small Request

If this book made a difference for you, even in a small way, would you consider leaving an honest review on Amazon or through the website you got a hold of this book?

As an independent author, I don't have the marketing budget of large publishing houses. Reviews are how readers discover books like this. Your feedback truly helps this work reach others who may need it.

It only takes a minute, and your honest thoughts, positive or critical are genuinely appreciated.

Scan the QR code below using your phone to leave your review.

Thank you for reading and for your support.

Closing Remark

You came to this program carrying something. Most people do. A hesitation on a kerb that did not used to be there. A hand that reached for the wall without being asked to. A quiet decision, made somewhere in the back of the mind, that certain things were better left untried.

That is where you started. What you have built across these four weeks is not the absence of that hesitation. It is something more durable than that. It is a nervous system that has been changed by practice. A body that has learned, through hundreds of deliberate repetitions, that movement can be trusted.

Ten minutes a day. Five days a week. That was the whole ask. And you did it.

The improvements you feel now, the greater steadiness on the standing leg, the heel that finds the floor with more confidence, the turn that no longer requires bracing, these are not the result of effort or willpower. They are the result of attention. Consistent, patient, daily attention to what the body is doing while it moves. That is a skill. And like all skills built on genuine repetition, it does not simply disappear when the four weeks end.

But it does require continuing.

Keep showing up. Keep moving slowly. Keep noticing. The ten minutes you have protected for this practice each week is not a small thing. It is a signal to your nervous system, your muscles, and your balance organs that they are needed, that they are being used, and that they should maintain themselves accordingly. The body responds to that signal every single time.

I have watched this change happen in hundreds of people across fifteen years of teaching. The student who took the stairs without thinking. The one who reached across the kitchen and felt nothing but steadiness. The one who walked to the end of the street and, halfway there, forgot to be afraid.

That moment of forgetting is the goal. Not the absence of risk, but the return of ease.

You have already taken the first steps. Keep going.

Acknowledgements

A book about the practice of moving together could not have been written alone.

My deepest gratitude goes to the hundreds of students I have had the privilege of teaching across fifteen years in community centers, rehabilitation facilities, and retirement homes. You taught me infinitely more than I taught you. Your resilience, your humor, your willingness to try something new in the most challenging seasons of your lives shaped every word of this program. This book exists because of what you showed me was possible.

To the physical therapists, occupational therapists, geriatric physicians, and healthcare professionals who generously shared their clinical expertise and trusted this practice enough to recommend it to their patients; your collaboration made this program safer, deeper, and more effective than it could ever have been without you.

To the global Tai Chi community whose devotion has preserved this art across generations, this book stands on your shoulders with respect.

To my colleagues in senior wellness who offered encouragement throughout this process, your support is reflected on every page.

To my own teachers who first placed these movements in my hands, I carry your instruction with me always.

Thank you. All of you.

— Xian Ming

About the Author

Xian Ming is a Certified Tai Chi and Qi Gong Instructor with a lifelong dedication to one purpose: helping older adults move better, live more freely, and age with confidence and dignity.

Over fifteen years of practice have taken Xian into community centers, retirement communities, and rehabilitation facilities, working directly with seniors navigating arthritis, chronic pain, balance challenges, anxiety, and mild cognitive decline. That depth of real-world experience shapes every page of this book.

Xian works in close collaboration with physical therapists, occupational therapists, and geriatric healthcare professionals to ensure every movement program meets the highest standards of safety and clinical relevance for older adults. This interdisciplinary approach has made Xian's chair-based Tai Chi and Qi Gong programs among the most trusted in senior wellness settings.

But beyond the credentials, what defines Xian's teaching is something simpler: a genuine belief that everybody, at every age, deserves a practice that meets it with patience, respect, and care.

Bonus: The 10-Minute Daily Quick Reference Guide

Feel free to print these pages, snap a picture of them with your smartphone, or simply lay it beside your practice space. Each week is a complete at-a-glance reference of what you need to do. This is everything you need without having to return to the chapter pages.

WEEK 1 PRACTICE – 10 Minutes Daily

Practice: 5 days per week | Rest: 2 days | Best time: Mid-morning (9–11 a.m.)

START: Three slow breaths. Feel all four corners of both feet on the floor.

Note: Column 1 (#) is the movement number of the actual movements as contained in chapters 6-9.

#	Movement	Illustration	Steps	What to Feel	Reps
1	**Rooted Stance**		① Feet hip-width · knees soft · crown lifts · shoulders drop ② Soften knees slightly · do not lock ③ Feel all four corners of each foot	Evenness across both feet · spine long without stiffness	3 breaths · use at start, close, and between every movement
2	**Empty Step** *(from Rooted Stance)*	*Shift weight left*	① Shift ALL weight onto one foot · feel it press into floor ② Only when fully transferred · lift free foot half an	Standing leg fully loaded · lifted foot completely weightless	4-6 cycles

#	Movement	Illustration	Steps	What to Feel	Reps
		Right foot empty & light	inch ③ Hold 2 sec · lower · shift to other side · repeat		
3	**Forward Walk** *(Empty Step set in motion)*	*Roll slowly from heel* *Transfer full weight to right foot*	① From Rooted Stance · perform Empty Step to free one foot ② Step it forward · HEEL lands first · roll slowly to toe ③ Transfer full weight to front foot before back foot lifts · continue	Heel contact before anything else · full roll from heel to toe · no hurrying	3-4 passes

#	Movement	Illustration	Steps	What to Feel	Reps
4	**Forward Walk + Arm Coord** *(continues Movement 3 · Day 3 onward only)*	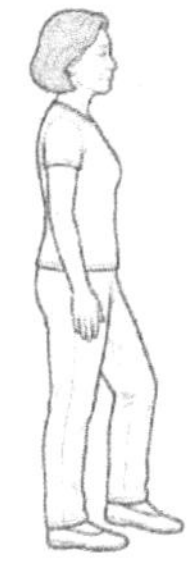 *Bring left foot forward* 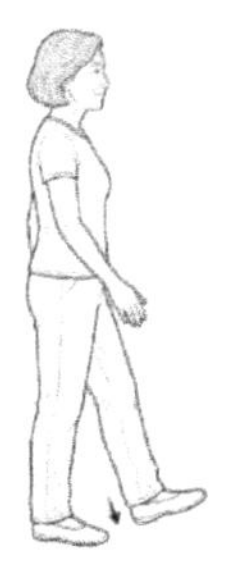 *Right foot forward, left arm forward, right arm backward* 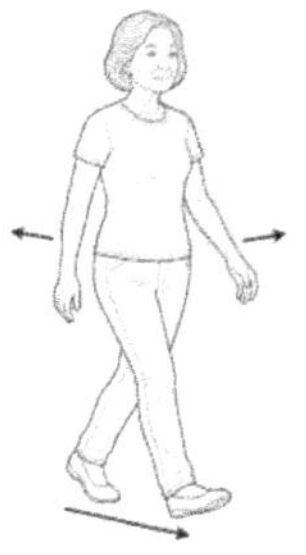 *Left foot forward, right arm forward, left arm backward*	① Walk exactly as Movement 3 · heel first · full weight transfer ② As right foot steps · left arm swings forward · right arm back and vice versa ③ Small swing · no higher than hip · hands relaxed and open	Cross-body coordination settling naturally after 2-3 steps · arms loose not forced	1-2 passes *(Day 3+ only)*

#	Movement	Illustration	Steps	What to Feel	Reps
		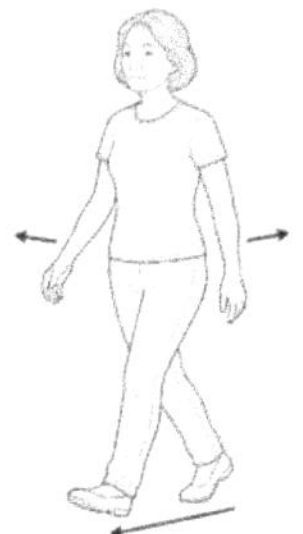			

CLOSE

#	Movement	Illustration	Steps	What to Feel	Reps
1	**Shoulder Rolls**		① Stand in Rooted Stance · arms hang loose ② Inhale · lift both shoulders toward ears ③ Exhale · roll backward in full circle · let them drop · repeat forward	Tension releasing from upper back and neck with each roll	× 2 backward · × 2 forward
2	**Ankle Circles** (*from Rooted Stance*)		① One hand lightly on wall for support ② Lift one foot one inch · rotate ankle in slow full circles ③ 4 rotations each direction · lower · repeat other side	Smooth continuous rotation · no stiffness	× 4 each direction · each ankle

#	Movement	Illustration	Steps	What to Feel	Reps
3	**Still Stand** *(from Rooted Stance)*		① Return to Rooted Stance · feet hip-width · knees soft ② Eyes softly closed or gaze lowered ③ Stand still · breathe naturally · notice feet now versus when you started	Quiet and settled · feet more present than at the start	60 seconds

Practice days this week — tick one per session:

☐ Day 1 ☐ Day 2 ☐ Day 3 ☐ Day 4 ☐ Day 5

Awkward is correct. Slow is correct. Show up, the foundation is being laid.

WEEK 2 PRACTICE – 10 Minutes Daily

Practice: 5 days per week | Rest: 2 days | Best time: Mid-morning (9–11 a.m.)

START: Three slow breaths. One breathe longer than Week 1.

Note: Column 1 (#) is the movement number of the actual movements as contained in chapters 6-9.

#	Movement	Illustration	Steps	What to Feel	Reps
1	**Rooted Stance**		① Feet hip-width · knees soft · four corners ② Let jaw unclench · let hands open	Settled and relaxed	3 breaths · use at start, close, and between every movement
2	**Empty Step** *(from Rooted Stance · same as Week 1)*	*See week 1 above*	① Shift ALL weight onto one foot ② Lift free foot · hold 2 sec · lower ③ Slower than Week 1 if possible · alternate sides	Complete transfer before any lift · standing leg solid	6 cycles
7	**Forward Walk + Arm Coord + Tai Chi Turn** *(continues Movement 4 from Week 1)*	*Weight shifts left from rooted stance after movement 4*	① Walk as Week 1 Movement 4 · heel first · opposite arm with each step ② At end of each pass · come to Rooted	Smooth and unhurried · arms resume naturally after each turn	2 passes · turn at each end

#	Movement	Illustration	Steps	What to Feel	Reps

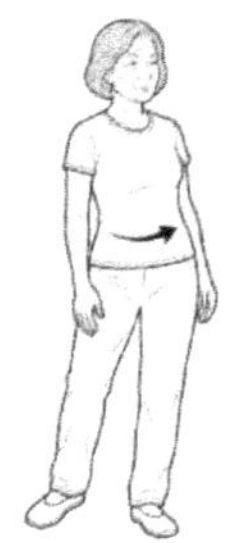

Lift and turn right foot at slight angle as weigh shifts right

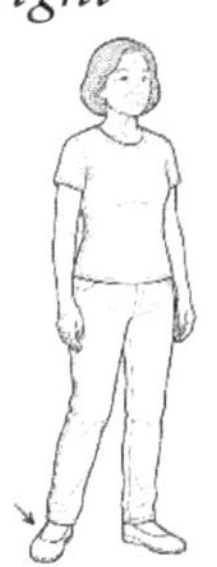

Empty left foot

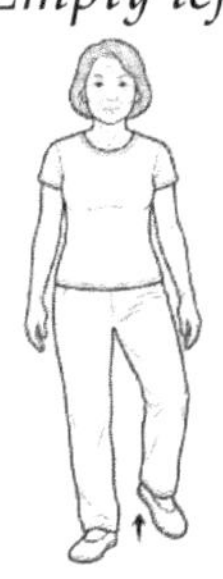

Bring left foot at rooted stance with right foot

Stance · arms settle
③ Tai Chi Turn · 2-3 small steps · weight shifts at every step · never pivot · resume walk with arms

#	Movement	Illustration	Steps	What to Feel	Reps
5	**Side Step** (*from Rooted Stance*)	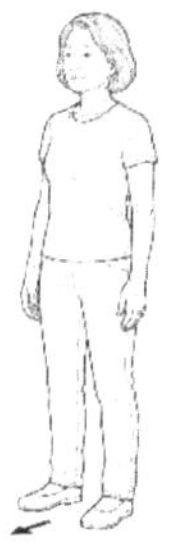 *Weight shifts left from rooted stance* 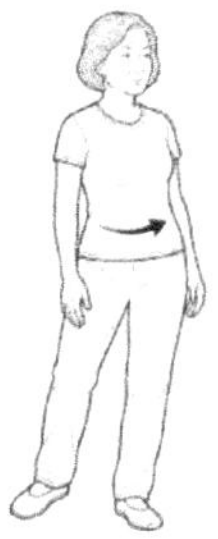 *Lift right foot slightly with right foot directly sideways* 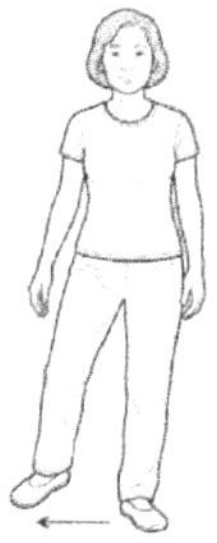 *Weight fully shifted to right foot and closed at hip width rooted stance*	① Shift full weight to one foot ② Step other foot directly sideways · whole sole lands flat · not heel or toe first ③ Shift weight fully to that foot · close first foot back to hip-width · pause · repeat both directions	Weight transfers fully before any foot lifts · stepping foot lands flat	3-4 steps each direction × 2 sets · one hand ON wall

#	Movement	Illustration	Steps	What to Feel	Reps
6	**Backward Step** *(from Rooted Stance)*	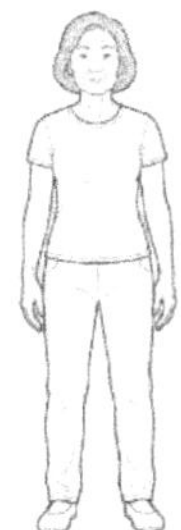 *Weight shifts right from rooted stance* 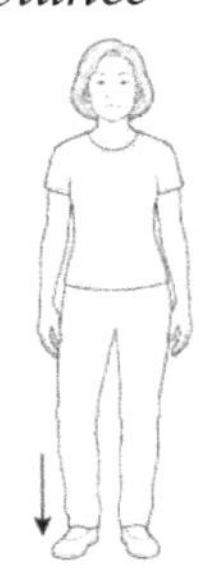 *Left foot backward, toes touch first* 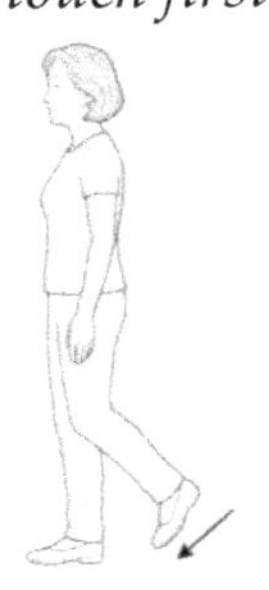 *Weight moved backward to left foot. Repeat backward for right foot*	① Check space behind before starting ② Shift weight to one foot · reach other foot backward · TOES touch first · lower heel ③ Transfer full weight back · spine stays upright · do not lean forward	Toes touching first clearly felt · spine upright not tilted forward	2 steps × 2-3 sequences · one hand ON wall

#	Movement	Illustration	Steps	What to Feel	Reps

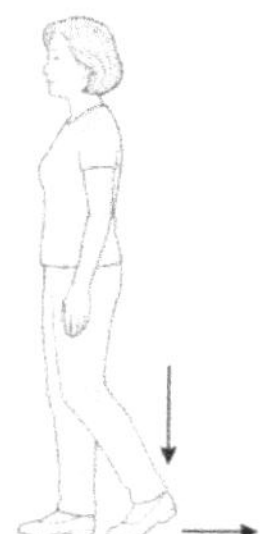

CLOSE: Follow the close session described in Week 1 Practice

Practice days this week — tick one per session:

☐ Day 1 ☐ Day 2 ☐ Day 3 ☐ Day 4 ☐ Day 5

Sideways and backward are new to the nervous system. Uncertainty means it is working.

WEEK 3 PRACTICE – 10 Minutes Daily

Practice: 5 days per week | Rest: 2 days | Best time: Mid-morning (9–11 a.m.)

START: Three slow breaths. Notice: is anything different from yesterday?

Note: Column 1 (#) is the movement number of the actual movements as contained in chapters 6-9.

#	Movement	Illustration	Steps	What to Feel	Reps
1	**Rooted Stance**		① Feet hip-width · knees soft · four corners ② Let jaw unclench · let hands open	Settled and relaxed	3 breaths · use at start, close, and between every movement
2	**Empty Step** *(from Rooted Stance · same as Week 2)*	*See week 1 above*	① Shift ALL weight onto one foot ② Lift free foot · hold 2 sec · lower ③ Alternate sides · slower than Week 2 if possible	Complete transfer · standing leg fully loaded	6 cycles
7	**Forward Walk + Arms + Tai Chi Turn** *(same as Week 2 Movement 7)*	*See week 2, movement 7*	① Walk heel first · opposite arm with each step ② Tai Chi Turn at each end · arms rest during turn · resume	More natural than Week 2 · less conscious effort needed	2 passes · turn at each end

#	Movement	Illustration	Steps	What to Feel	Reps
			immediately after ③ No change from Week 2 · let it feel more settled		
8	**Cloud Hands Walking** *(continues directly from Movement 7's arm swing · do not stop between)*	*Right arm raises, shoulder height & right foot forward; left arm lowers toward hip & left foot backward.* *Repeat arm and leg movement on opposite side*	① At the end of movement 7's final forward walk pass · do not stop · let the arm swing slow and widen ② One arm rises toward shoulder height as the other lowers toward hip · palms alternate facing in and out ③ Arms and legs move together · rotation comes from relaxation · not effort	Fluid not mechanical · one moment where arm and leg move as one thing	4-6 steps × 2-3 passes
9	**Controlled High Step** *(frcm Rooted Stance)*	*From rooted stance, shift weight to left foot*	① Shift full weight to standing foot · feel it press firmly into	Standing leg presses firmly · lifting leg completely	4--6 steps × 2 passes · one hand on wall

#	Movement	Illustration	Steps	What to Feel	Reps
		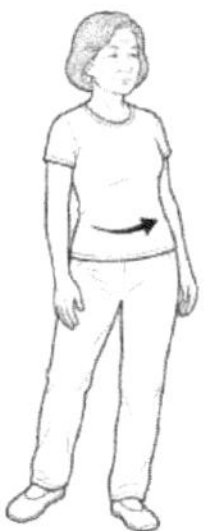 *Lift right knee* 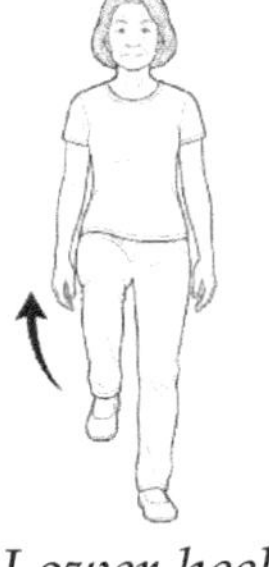 *Lower heel in forward walk; repeat on opposite leg* 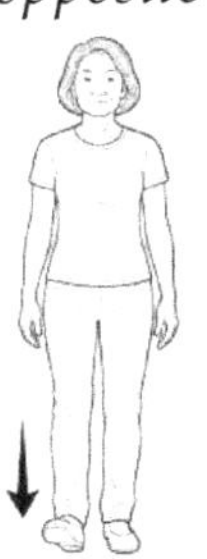	floor ② Slowly lift opposite knee to comfortable height · pause briefly · foot hangs relaxed ③ Lower heel first exactly as Forward Walk · shift weight forward · continue	relaxed · heel lands first	
10	**Tandem Walk** (*from Rooted Stance*)	*From rooted stance with left hand on wall*	① Step one foot forward · place it directly in front of the other · heel close to toes ② Shift full weight onto	Narrow base clearly felt · less precarious by Day 5 than Day 1	4--6 steps × 2 passes

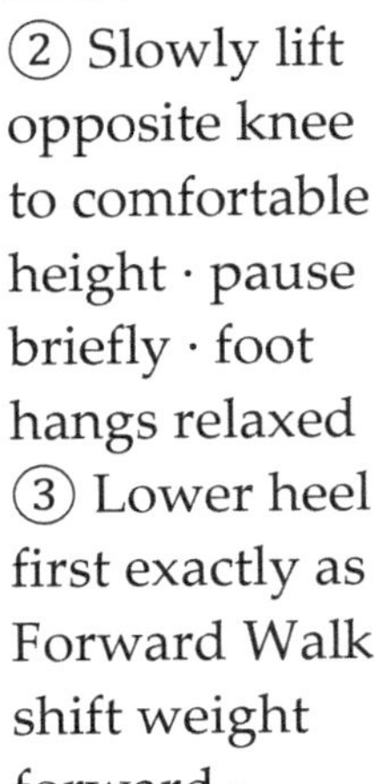

#	Movement	Illustration	Steps	What to Feel	Reps
		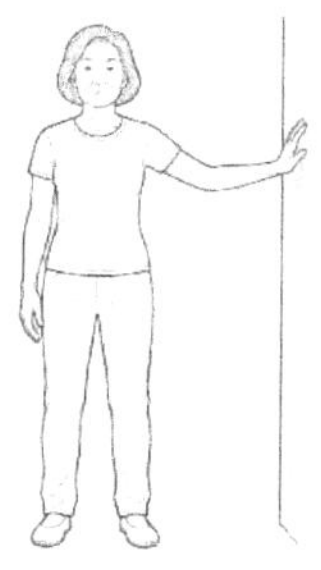 *Right foot in front of left foot (heel-toe); shift weight right* 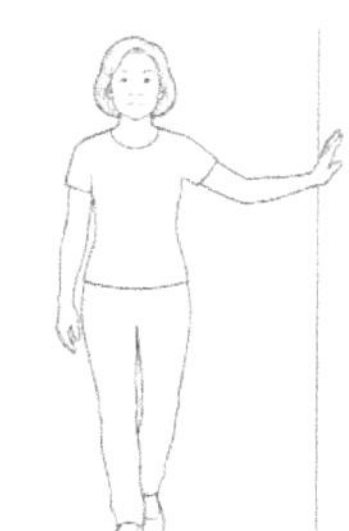 *Left foot in front of right foot (heel-toe); shift weight left* 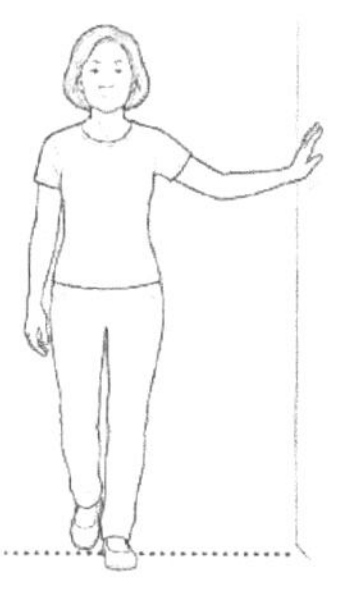	front foot · step other foot forward in the same way ③ Gaze straight ahead · not at feet · wall within fingertip reach throughout		
5 & 6	**Side Step +** **Backward** **Step** (*review* ·	*See week 2, movement 5&6*	Review only · perform exactly as Week 2 · 1	Both directions feeling more	1 set each direction

#	Movement	Illustration	Steps	What to Feel	Reps
	same as Week 2)		set each · skip if session feels full	reliable than Week 2	

CLOSE: Follow the close session described in Week 1 Practice

Practice days this week — tick one per session:

☐ Day 1 ☐ Day 2 ☐ Day 3 ☐ Day 4 ☐ Day 5

What felt separate is starting to feel like one thing. Stay with the slowness.

WEEK 4 PRACTICE – 10 Minutes Daily

Practice: 5 days per week | Rest: 2 days | Best time: Mid-morning (9–11 a.m.)

Outdoor Practice (Days 3–5): One session may be done outdoors on a flat quiet surface. Same flat-soled shoes as indoors. Let the environment settle before you begin. Same pace as indoors. The variability of the ground is the training.

START: Three slow breaths. One longer exhale. Notice one thing different from Week 1.

Note: Column 1 (#) is the movement number of the actual movements as contained in chapters 6-9.

#	Movement	Illustration	Steps	What to Feel	Reps
1	**Rooted Stance**		① Feet hip-width · knees soft · four corners ② Crown lifts · tailbone drops · shoulders release	Settled · this is not a warm-up · this is the practice beginning	3 breaths · use at start, close, and between every movement
2	**Empty Step** *(from Rooted Stance · same as Week 1)*	*See week 1 above*	① Shift ALL weight onto one foot · lift · hold 2 sec · lower ② Alternate sides · unhurried · this is the practice not a warm-up	Standing leg solid · lifted foot weightless	6 cycles

#	Movement	Illustration	Steps	What to Feel	Reps
3, 7, 8, 9	**Forward Walk → Cloud Hands** *(Movements 3, 7, 8, 9 combined into one flowing sequence)*	*See movements 3,7,8 and 9 in week 1, week 2 and week 3 above*	① Passes 1-2: walk heel first with standard arm swing · Tai Chi Turn at each end ② Passes 3-4: let arm swing drift naturally into Cloud Hands as you walk ③ Weave one Controlled High Step naturally into each pass ④ Let transitions between walk and Cloud Hands happen · do not force them	Everything beginning to feel like one continuous movement rather than separate steps	4 passes total
5	**Side Steps** *(from Rooted Stance · same as previous weeks)*	*See week 2, movement 5*	① Shift weight fully to one foot · step other foot sideways · whole sole lands flat ② Shift weight fully to that foot · close first foot back to hip-	Weight shift feeling more automatic than Week 2	4 steps each direction × 2 sets

#	Movement	Illustration	Steps	What to Feel	Reps
			width ③ Repeat both directions		
6	**Backward Steps** (*from Rooted Stance · same as previous weeks*)	*See week 2, movement 6*	① Check behind · shift weight to one foot · reach other foot back · toes first ② Lower heel · transfer weight fully · spine upright ③ 2 steps · pause in Rooted Stance · repeat	Spine upright and confident · toes landing first without thinking	3 sequences
10	**Tandem Walk** (*from Rooted Stance · continues Week 3 Movement 10*)	*See week 3, movement 10*	① Heel to toe · one foot directly in front of the other ② Gaze forward · not at feet · wall nearby throughout ③ Day 3 onward: attempt one pass without touching wall	Narrow base manageable · gaze staying forward naturally	2 passes

CLOSE: Follow the close session described in Week 1 Practice

Practice days this week — tick one per session:

☐ Day 1 ☐ Day 2 ☐ Day 3 ☐ Day 4 ☐ Day 5

No new movements. Only the practice, finally flowing as one thing.